Tough Questions, Great Answers

Tough Questions, Great Answers

Responding to Patient Concerns about Today's Dentistry

Robin Wright, MA

quintessence
books

Quintessence Publishing Co, Inc
Chicago, Berlin, London, Tokyo, Paris, Barcelona,
São Paulo, Moscow, Prague, and Warsaw

Library of Congress Cataloging-in-Publication Data

Wright, Robin, MA.
    Tough questions, great answers : responding to patient concerns about today's dentistry / Robin Wright.
       p.   cm.
    Includes bibliographical references and index.
    ISBN 0-86715-320-2
    1. Dentistry—Psychological aspects.   2. Dentist and patient.
I. Title.
    [DNLM: 1. Dentist–Patient Relations.   2. Dentistry.
3. Communication.   WU 61 W952t 1997]
RK53.W74 1997
617.6′023—dc21   97-19573
for Library of Congress   CIP

quintessence
books

©1997 by Quintessence Publishing Co, Inc

Quintessence Publishing Co, Inc
551 N. Kimberly Drive
Carol Stream, IL 60188-1881

Editor: Patricia Bereck Weikersheimer
Production/Design: Lisa Ream
Printing and Binding: Carlith Printing Inc, Illinois, USA

Contents

Acknowledgments

My appreciation goes to the talented dental professionals who, by participating in my research and seminars, helped create many of the great answers in this book. And special thanks to my expert panel for their extraordinary efforts in reviewing the manuscript: Ginny Thiersch, Washington, DC; Katherine Rowan, PhD, Purdue University; Brenda Eustice, RN, Peoria, Illinois; Richard Price, DMD, Newton, Massachusetts; and Richard Smith, DDS, Atlanta, Georgia.

Special Note

A word about how the "Q & A" sections throughout the book are organized: Some patient questions are followed immediately by a suggested "great answer," other questions are followed by a "possible answer." The "possible answers" were submitted by your colleagues around the country as the responses they now use with patients. This eavesdropping is often interesting, sometimes humorous, but always educational. An analysis of the effective and ineffective parts of a possible response is an excellent way to develop an even better answer.

If you wish to provide the author with tough patient questions to be addressed in any future editions of this book, access http://www.greatanswers.com.

Introduction

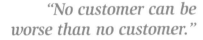

Patients ask: "Why does dentistry cost so much?" "Do you guarantee your work?" "Do you treat AIDS patients?" "If it didn't hurt before treatment, why does it hurt now?" "If X-rays are so safe, why do you leave the room when you take them?" "Why didn't my previous hygienist say anything about gum disease?" "Why did my insurance company say you are too expensive?"

You face tough questions from patients in your practice. Your success in communication is most critical—and most difficult—when a patient voices a challenging question or concern. Many dental professionals say, "I'm an effective communicator when the patient is predictable and pleasant. I'm not as effective when the patient is troublesome. If the patient pitches them underhanded, I'm fine. But what do I say when the patient plays hardball?" By focusing on specific tough questions, this book targets the skills most required for full communication competence in a dental practice.

Great Answers = Technical Knowledge + Communication Skills

When you get a tough patient question, you usually know far more about the subject—be it insurance, post-treatment medication, or office policy—than you have time to tell. Unfortunately, knowing even a hundred possible answers to any given question does not lead automatically to choosing the right one for a particular patient situation.

I once asked an orthopedic surgeon in a media interview, "Why are some patients so dissatisfied with their orthopedic surgeons?" He answered, "Well, I know of one doctor who was sued for cutting off the wrong leg." Why did he choose that particular message out of his vast array of knowledge? He could have said, "When a patient is dissatisfied, it's usually not a lack of care, but a lack of understanding between the patient and the doctor. Through communication, concerns can be resolved. So if you are unhappy with any aspect of your treatment, call your doctor—not your lawyer—first."

I was waiting at an airport gate to board a flight when the airline representative announced, "This flight has been delayed due to mechanical difficulty with the aircraft. Because this is a new type of aircraft, the mechanics are not sure they can repair it." Of all the information the airline representative had about the situation, she chose to inform her passengers that the mechanics were unsure of their abilities. (In other words, we would be hurled at great speed, thousands of feet above the ground, in a vehicle no one knew how to fix.) Far better if she had said, "Either this aircraft will be restored to perfect working condition or a different aircraft will be provided for your flight."

Seeing a dentist in a face mask for the first time, I asked, "Are you wearing that mask because you have a cold?" He replied, "I'm not wearing this mask to protect you from me. I'm wearing it to protect me from you." The dentist could have strengthened, rather than sabotaged, the relationship by describing how infection control procedures effectively serve to protect patients from the transmission of disease.

Great answers require more than technical knowledge on a topic. Great answers demand communication skills to guide you in selecting what dental information to share in response to a particular patient's concern.

Good Communication Leads to Practice Success

Although clinical skill is essential to practice success, it isn't enough. A strong practice is built by "doing good and telling about it." If you are like many dental professionals, your treatment is better than your talk about treatment. Here are four reasons why effective communication is important to your practice.

Reason 1: Patients assess clinical excellence by communication style

Because dentistry is a service, not a product, it is intangible. Little of dental care can be seen, held, sampled, or returned if unsuitable. Therefore, the patient cannot judge the quality of your service except by the way in which it is delivered. Any interaction with a patient can become a "moment of truth," defined as a point at which a patient forms an impression (accurate or inaccurate) of the quality of care you provide.[1]

Because patients cannot judge accurately the quality of clinical treatment, they fill this uncomfortable vacuum in judgment by assessing nonclinical aspects of your care. For example, your treatment methods may be judged as up-to-date as your reception room furniture. If a patient worried about fluoride is told, "Fluoride isn't toxic in the dosage of your fluoride treatment, but don't swallow it," she will not be particularly reassured. If a patient hears from a staff member, "The treatment is expensive, isn't it?" he may doubt the fairness of your fees. Patients often say "yes" or "no" based upon the communication they have with you or your team.

Reason 2: Patient satisfaction is based on communication

Health-care research proves patient satisfaction is created largely by the communication skill of the health-care provider.[2,3,4] Conversely, poor communication is the most common reason for dissatisfaction with care and for a decision to terminate the doctor-patient relationship.[5,6] Personal contact with you and your team, whether positive or negative, is the most memorable aspect of dental care for patients.[7]

Reason 3: Patients aren't telling you everything

Although some days it seems like the appointment book is packed with patients bent on making "mountains out of molehills" and "tempests in teapots," patients actually want more communication with you than they are willing to ask for. Research shows that patients are reluctant to raise questions, ask for information, or voice their important concerns to their doctors.[4,8,9] A full 45 percent of patient concerns and 54 percent of patient complaints are not elicited by physicians.[10] Further, patients who ask direct questions end up more satisfied in their communication with health-care professionals than patients who ask indirect questions.[11]

Reason 4: Patients walk even if they don't talk

Although patients may not voice their complaints, they will still leave your practice if they are dissatisfied. Patients don't always tell you about the source of their dissatisfaction, but they do tell the neighborhood. Consider these findings in a 1991 national public opinion study from the Gallup Organization, commissioned by the American Dental Association:[12]

- 60 percent of dental patients said they would change dentists if they were dissatisfied or had a problem
- 23 percent said they would talk with their dentist to resolve a problem
- 90 percent said they would tell family and friends about their dissatisfaction with the dental practice

A referral from family and friends is the way most consumers find a dentist. Satisfied patients are the leading source of new business—and dissatisfied patients are a threat to practice growth.

Communication Benefits

When you communicate effectively, patients tend to:

- Experience less anxiety
- Experience less discomfort
- Require less medication
- Recuperate more quickly
- Stay with the practice
- Remember and follow instructions
- Pay their bills on time
- Refer other patients to the practice
- Be less likely to sue

Good Communication Benefits Your Patients and Your Practice

A classic study in health-care research shows that good communication between doctors and patients can lead to less postoperative pain, less medication, and earlier recovery.[13] Other research suggests that good communication increases patient utilization of dental services and inhibits patient anxiety.[14] Patients are more likely to comply with recommended treatment if they have a strong respect for the dentist and staff.[15] Patients who have a good relationship with their health-care providers are more likely to remember and follow instructions, refer other patients, and pay their bills than patients who have a less positive relationship with their health-care providers.[16] Finally, patients who are satisfied with their doctors are less likely to sue.[17]

Get Ready for Real Patient Questions

This book isn't built on hypothetical situations. It is based on what dental teams say are the most difficult questions facing them in the delivery of dental care, according to my research with U.S. dental practices during the last four years. The questions fell into the following categories:

- **Trust:** Building confidence in the doctor's skill and judgment
- **Safety:** Reassuring patients of the safety of dental treatment
- **Motivation:** Gaining understanding, agreement, and action on dental treatment
- **Cost:** Explaining dental fees, benefit coverage, and managed care plans
- **Reception:** Managing patient concerns about office policies

Patient Questions

Themes	Communication goals
Can I trust you?	Build patient confidence in the doctor's skill and judgment
Am I safe here?	Reassure patients about treatment safety
Is the treatment worth it?	Motivate patients to accept needed treatment
Why does it cost so much?	Effectively explain cost and dental benefits
Why do you have that policy?	Protect patient relationships in reception

Good Communicators Need More than Scripted Answers

You've no doubt noticed that this book contains more than just great answers to tough questions. It features ways to diagnose patient concerns and treat them through effective communication. There is no "magic bullet" in dentistry or communication. A single procedure can't fix every dental problem; a single answer won't work with every patient. Just as you need to analyze a patient's total health to recommend an ideal dental treatment, so you need to analyze a communication situation to implement an ideal approach in your answer to a particular patient's question.

The next two chapters get you off to a good start in communication by explaining how to discover the patient's true concerns and how to begin your answers to tough questions. The rest of the book is organized around the previously described categories of questions. Each chapter presents central goals, common obstacles, and the necessary skills for addressing a particular type of communication challenge.

Chapter 1 "'What's Going On?' Encouraging Communication in Patient Interviews" examines effective patient interview techniques and offers tips for good listening.

Chapter 2 "'Do You Care?' Starting a Successful Answer" suggests how to (and how not to) begin your answers to tough patient questions.

Chapter 3 "'Are You Any Good?' Building Trust in the Doctor's Skill and Judgment" gives communication techniques to build patient trust in the dentist's abilities. You will find questions and answers related to patient confidence in the dental practice.

Chapter 4 "'Am I Safe?' Reassuring Patients of Treatment Safety" analyzes how to respond effectively to patient concerns about safety issues. It gives positive messages for patient questions about infection control, X-rays, amalgam, fluoride, and water lines.

Chapter 5 "'Is It Worth It?' Motivating Patients to Accept Treatment" tells how to be clear, concise, and caring when educating patients about clinical aspects of treatment. It describes how to make effective case presentations, overcome patient objections to treatment, and encourage patient compliance with post-treatment instructions.

Chapter 6 "'It Costs How Much?' Explaining Fees and Dental Benefits" discusses how patients perceive dental costs, gives practical tips on talking to patients about money, and provides answers to questions about fees, dental benefits, and managed care plans.

Chapter 7 "'What's the Policy?' Protecting Patient Relationships in Reception" gives practical communication guidelines for receptionists, with specific questions and answers for reception room contact.

Chapter 8 "Communication Goals for the Dental Team" offers communication job descriptions for each member of the dental team.

Loan This Book to Everyone on Your Team

Receptionists and practice administrators: You field questions on the telephone about every aspect of the practice from fees to the dentist's qualifications. You get tough questions at the front desk about appointment scheduling and office policies. You will benefit from all the material, but Chapter 7 is dedicated to your particular communication concerns.

Dental assistants: You sit in the hot seat when the patient says, "I hated to mention this to the doctor, but . . . " You are challenged by the need to build patient trust, reduce patient anxiety, summarize the doctor's recommendations, and overcome patient objections to treatment. You will find Chapters 2 through 5 especially helpful.

Hygienists: You are faced with explaining hard-to-understand clinical concepts and motivating patients to follow home-care instructions. Chapters 2 and 5 are most relevant to your communication challenges.

Business managers: You will find Chapter 6 most valuable on responding to tough questions about dental fees and insurance coverage. Because you encounter treatment objections during financial discussions, you will find Chapter 5 on treatment motivation helpful as well.

Dentists and dental students: You will find every chapter relevant for making positive personal contact with patients and guiding your dental team's communication on difficult patient issues. As the arbiter of practice policy, you give the final "thumbs up" or "thumbs down" to every answer suggested in this book.

A Game Plan to Enhance Communication

As you read the book, mark the pages that have answers you find effective. (You might color-code the marked pages by team member, perhaps placing red paper clips on the pages for the appointment coordinator, green for the dental assistant, and so on.) Then, the following eight R's of communication change will help you gain full value from this book.

Research

Find out the tough questions that face your dental practice in particular. Ask each team member to complete the work sheet on page 10. Request team members to bring their completed work sheets to a staff meeting in two weeks.

Review

Use the staff meeting to review the tough patient questions and current answers in your practice. Discuss for each: Does the current response meet the needs of the patient? Does it present a desired image for the practice? Would such supporting materials as booklets or visuals make communication easier?

Revise

Working individually or as a team, prepare revised answers to your tough patient questions. Use and edit the suggested answers in this book. Check your revised answers:

- Is it clear?
- Is it accurate?
- Is it brief?
- Does it meet the patient's need for information?
- Does it demonstrate empathy and caring?
- Does it present a positive image of the practice?

Record

A permanent record will serve as a helpful refresher for current staff and a valuable training tool for new staff. As a format for your permanent record, use a set of index cards with a question and answer on each card. (These cards can be prepared easily by using the postcard format on your word-processing software.) The cards will be a handy reference when placed in a drawer at the front desk and in the treatment rooms.

Rehearse

Refine the answers and sharpen your personal communication style by practicing the responses. Using a videotape or audiotape to record and review practice sessions brings the quickest change in communication behavior.

Respond

You will receive a fair return on your investment of time only if you actually use the answers. Ignore the butterflies in your stomach and try that new answer in a patient conversation. If an approach is especially effective, be sure to tell your team members.

Reward

When your new behaviors in communication receive positive patient response, reward yourself and your staff. If new behaviors still need work, reward yourselves anyway. You will enhance commitment to the process of communication change.

Rework

Patient concerns change with the health-care environment. Research, review, and rework patient communication materials once a year.

Dental Team Work Sheet

We hope to solve the communication challenges you face in our practice. Please help by filling out this brief questionnaire. What are three of the toughest questions patients ask you? What's your favorite answer? Please phrase questions and answers as "true to life" as possible.

Question: _____
_____
_____

Answer: _____
_____
_____
_____
_____

Question: _____
_____
_____

Answer: _____
_____
_____
_____
_____

Question: _____
_____
_____

Answer: _____
_____
_____
_____
_____

Comments: _____
_____
_____
_____
_____

Please bring this work sheet with you to our next staff meeting.

Skill Summary

- As a skilled dental professional, you communicate successfully with the majority of your patients. A focus on difficult patient encounters targets the skills you need most for full communication competence in dental practice.

- Patient perceptions of quality care are created more by your communication competence than by your clinical ability.

- Encouraging patients to voice their concerns must be a priority for your practice. Most patients want more communication from you than they are willing to ask for. Further, many patients will leave a dental practice if dissatisfied, but few will tell the practice about the source of their dissatisfaction.

- To present a positive image of your practice, work with your dental team to anticipate difficult patient questions and prepare effective responses to patient concerns.

References

1. Albrecht K, Zemke R. Service America! Homewood, IL: Dow Jones-Irwin Publishers; 1985.

2. Thompson TL. Patient health care: Issues in interpersonal communication. In Ray EB, Donohew L (eds): Communication and Health: Systems and Applications. Hillsdale, NJ: Lawrence Earlbaum; 1990:27–44.

3. DiMatteo MR. A social-psychological analysis of physician-patient rapport: Toward a science of the art of medicine. Journal of Social Issues 1979;35:12–33.

4. Daly MB, Hulka BS. Talking with the Doctor, 2. Journal of Communication 1975;25:148–152.

5. Hall JA, Roter DL, Katz NR. Meta-analysis of correlates of provider behavior in medical encounters. Medical Care 1988;26:657–675.

6. Kasteler J, Kane RL, Olsen DM, Thetford C. Issues underlying prevalence of "doctor-shopping" behavior. Journal of Health and Social Behavior 1976; 17:328–339.

7. Ruben BD. The health caregiver–patient relationship: Pathology, etiology, treatment. In Ray BR, Donohew L (eds): Communication and Health: Systems and Applications. Hillsdale, NJ: Lawrence Earlbaum; 1990:51–68.

8. Adler K. Doctor-patient communication: A shift to problem-oriented research. Human Communication Research 1977;3:179–190.

9. Korsch BM, Negrete VF. Doctor-patient communication. Scientific American 1972;227:66–74.

10. Stewart MA, McWhinney IR, Buch CW. The doctor-patient relationship and its effect upon outcome. Journal of the Royal College of General Practitioners 1979;27:77–81.

11. Roter DL. Patient question-asking in physician-patient interaction. Health Psychology 1984;3:395–409.

12. Dentistry in the 90's: Consumer Attitudes and How They Affect Your Practice. Department of Marketing and Seminar Services. Chicago: American Dental Association; 1991.

13. Egbert LD, Battit GE, Welch CE, Bartlett MK. Reduction in post-operative pain by encouragement and instruction of patients: A study of doctor-patient rapport. New Eng J Med 1964;270:825–827.

14. Corah NL, O'Shea RM, Bissell GD. The dentist-patient relationship: Perceptions by patients of dental behavior in relation to satisfaction and anxiety. JADA 1985;111:443–446.

15. Jepsen CH. Some behavioral aspects of dental patient compliance. Journal of Dental Practice Administration 1986;3(4):117–122.

16. Bates RC. The Fine Art of Understanding Patients. Oradell, NJ: Medical Economics; 1968.

17. Medical Malpractice. Washington, DC: Department of Health, Education and Welfare; 1973.

"What's Going On?"

Encouraging Communication in Patient Interviews

"If the physician will listen, the patient will tell the diagnosis."

—Sir William Osler

Only when you know a patient's perspective can you build a positive relationship. Only when you know a patient's needs can you recommend treatment. Only when you know a patient's desires can you influence the acceptance of ideal dental care. Your communication goals—good relationships, case acceptance, and patient satisfaction—all begin with knowing your patients. As Dr. L.D. Pankey advised, "Never treat a stranger."

Quality Care and Patient Satisfaction Come When Patients Talk to You

By encouraging patients to talk to you and your team, you build trust and reduce patient anxiety.[1] You enhance satisfaction with the doctor-patient relationship, and thus strengthen satisfaction with your practice.[2,3]

Open communication influences not only your relationship with patients, it influences quality of care. Communication is key to patient assessment. Patient assessment is key to treatment planning. Therefore, patient communication is crucial to the provision of appropriate dental care. Your ability to ask questions—and listen to the answers—determines the amount and accuracy of information you obtain from patients. If you are successful at getting patients to talk, they will offer key facts about their dental condition and medical history. Equally important, they will tell you what they really want in dentistry.

Thus, encouraging communication is a first step in persuasion. Dr. Omar Reed notes that people buy not because they understand but because they feel understood.[4] A patient who feels rushed through an "assembly line" dental office may refuse treatment. Conversely, a patient who receives an attentive ear from a doctor is more likely to accept treatment and less likely to reschedule or cancel appointments.[5] Every time a patient tells you something, you get a clue for motivating that patient to say "yes" to treatment.

A dentist once asked me why some two-minute problems take two-hour visits. Are time constraints the down side to encouraging patient communication? Actually, listening can save time in the long run. For example, a patient's description of his or her health condition usually takes less than two and a half minutes.[6] If the patient is interrupted, he will restate his concerns at the end of the visit. Because these concerns are often significant, the visit must be lengthened to accommodate them.

Why Encourage Patients to Talk?

Helps patients discover their dental needs and preferences
Clarifies patients' understanding of dental problems
Builds trust in the doctor-patient relationship
Decreases missed appointments
Reduces patient anxiety
Persuades patients to accept needed care
Encourages patients to take a more active role in their dental health
Motivates patients to follow treatment instructions
Increases patient satisfaction

Report Card: Do Doctors Make the Grade on Promoting Communication?

Unfortunately, many health-care professionals get low marks on encouraging patients to talk. As a result, they miss out on information central to accurate diagnoses, treatment acceptance, and patient satisfaction. In receiving health care, patients have a desire for information but do not necessarily demand it. Not only are patients reluctant to raise concerns, but health-care providers are reluctant to listen to them. According to research, 25 to 50 percent of patients do not mention their health worries to their doctors because of a lack of opportunity or encouragement.[2,7,8] Other research shows that patients discuss their medical concerns for an average of 18 seconds before they are interrupted by health-care providers.[9]

A Hidden Agenda: To Know the Answer, First Know the Question

Just as knowing the patient leads to the best treatment recommendation, so knowing the question leads to the best answer. But sometimes a patient's question is ambiguous. The true concern may be hidden in generalities, cloaked in humor, or concealed in an off-hand remark. To complicate matters further, a spoken question may not prompt the same answer as the hidden question behind it.

A patient once asked, "Do you treat AIDS patients?" The dentist answered, "We just don't know. First, patients do not always include everything on their medical history. Second, people can be HIV-positive and not know it. So there's no way to tell if we are treating an HIV carrier or not." I later asked the patient what her concerns were—and whether the dentist had answered them. She stated, "I wanted to know if I was safe from getting AIDS here and the doctor said he didn't know. I'm more worried now than I was before I asked the question."

Because the dentist missed the patient's hidden question, he missed the opportunity to provide a reassurance of safety. Two essential skills allow you to diagnose a patient's true dental concerns: effective listening and interviewing.

Listening Skills: Stay on Track by Avoiding the Roadblocks to Communication

It's been said that an open ear is the only believable sign of an open heart. Unfortunately, most people are just not good listeners. They remember only half of what they hear immediately after a conversation. Within 48 hours they forget a full 75 percent.[10] In one study,[11] students in a lecture course recorded their thoughts when a buzzer sounded at random intervals during the semester. Only 12 percent were listening to the lecture at any given time. Sex was the thought of choice for 20 percent of the students. Others were reminiscing, worrying, daydreaming, and the like. The average person doesn't follow Shakespeare's advice to "give every man thy ear, but few thy voice."

Six Roadblocks to Good Listening

Office distractions
Mental vacations
Personal bias
Diagnostic facts
Frequent interruptions
Patient distractions

The following suggests ways to help you truly hear a patient's story and become a better listener.

Protect yourself from office distractions

A party guest once greeted his distracted hostess by saying, "I'm sorry I'm late, but I murdered my wife earlier this evening and had the toughest time stuffing her body into the trunk of my car." The hostess smiled and said, "Well, darling, the important thing is that you've arrived, and now my party can really begin."

No one listens well when preoccupied with other matters. Do you flip through professional journals while on the phone with patients? Do you ask a patient how she is while washing your hands, checking the instrument tray, or reviewing her chart? How frequently are you interrupted by office matters during patient conversations? Do you need to revise your office policy on taking telephone calls during dental visits? Review the demands of your practice routine to set aside ample listening time for patients.

Avoid mental vacations

Suppose you ordered black coffee in a restaurant, and the waitress asked, "Cream and sugar?" You would know her body was at your table, but her mind was far away. People can listen about four times faster than they can talk. Many use this extra time to take mental vacations. You can stay on track by mentally summarizing the patient's message or listening for central concerns underlying surface remarks.

Beware of bias

A training course for police officers was disrupted when a woman waving a banana chased a man across the back of the room. (Makes dental meetings seem staid, doesn't it?) Asked to describe what they had just seen, many of the attendees gave inaccurate reports. They said the man was chasing the woman, and the banana became a gun. This interpretation of events more closely matched the *expectations* of the police officers.

Most people tend to see what they expect to see and hear what they expect to hear. If you know that people tend to slant messages to agree with their attitudes, you can protect yourself from this unwanted listening bias.

You also need to beware of listening in "black and white" instead of "shades of gray," thus reacting strongly to a negative word or phrase. For example, if a patient said in an initial interview that he wanted "cheap dentistry," you wouldn't adjust your treatment recommendations based on just one comment. Or, if a patient seemed indifferent about preventing gum disease, you wouldn't assume that she was equally indifferent about all other aspects of her oral health and appearance.

Listen for more than just facts

At the end of a long day, it's tempting to listen only for facts relevant to diagnosis and treatment planning. Instead, listen for central themes, underlying opinions, and dental priorities as well as diagnostic facts. These important cues can help you frame treatment recommendations in the patient's language.

Don't interrupt

Lincoln was once asked how he managed to listen effectively to widely differing points of view. He answered, "I find it helps to stop talking." To protect your schedule (and your sanity), it's tempting to interrupt or finish the patient's sentences. It's tempting to plan your response while the patient is talking. However, these conversational habits show that you are not listening at peak effectiveness. Listening experts recommend that you listen more than you talk, refrain from interrupting, and hold writing on the chart to a minimum.

Overcome patient distractions

An unusual haircut, a unique style of clothing, or a different speaking style can be far more interesting than what the patient is saying. Such questions as "Who is his barber?" or "What's that accent?" can make you miss valuable clues to the patient's point of view. Focus on the patient's message instead of distracting aspects of appearance or speaking style.

Body Language That Says "I'm Listening"

Try	Avoid
Making consistent eye contact	Looking away as you or the patient speaks
Positioning yourself at an equal level with the patient	Standing over the patient; standing while the patient sits
Nodding and smiling as the patient speaks	Having little change in facial expressions; showing negative reactions
Having a relaxed but erect posture	Slouching or an unusually stiff posture
Leaning forward in your chair	Leaning back in your chair
Positioning your body toward the patient	Positioning your body away from the patient
Keeping an open upper body position	Folding your arms
Using gestures that complement your message	Fidgeting, shuffling papers, or covering your mouth or eyes

Interviewing Skills: Get a Complete Picture of Patient Concerns

When you observe a patient in an initial interview, you assess his dental condition in particular and his personality in general. This judgment guides your conversation, influences the care you recommend, and ultimately determines your relationship with the patient.[12] Since patient assessment is so important to quality care and quality relationships, you must do it well. How can you efficiently employ the communication tools for interviewing to get a complete and accurate picture of the patient's perspective?

Tool 1: Open questions

An open question is one that gives great freedom in the choice of an answer. It does not guide or limit the response except in terms of the topic. Sample open questions are: "What was it like?," "What did you notice about it?," and "How did you feel about that?" Open questions will tell you what the patient already knows, what the patient thinks is important, and how the patient feels about a dental topic. Open questions show respect and create comfort. Unfortunately, they also consume time. Use open questions to begin an interview and to introduce a new topic in an interview.

Good questions to begin the patient interview
- How can I help you?
- What brings you to our office?
- It's great to see you, Ms. Anderson. What particular reason do you have for today's visit?

Bad questions to begin the patient interview
- Did you fill out the medical/dental history form?
- What's your dental problem?
- Why are you here?

When patients don't respond to open questions, perhaps they
- Aren't sure how much detail you need
- Aren't sure what kind of answer you want
- Don't understand the question
- Don't know the answer
- Knew the answer but have forgotten it
- Feel the question is irrelevant (or none of your business)

Follow-up strategies for open questions help patients tell their stories.

Tool 2: Facilitations and Probes

Facilitations are short remarks that let the patient know you are listening. They encourage the patient to tell you more. Probes encourage patients to give more specific information on a particular subject. Use them when you suspect a patient has not shared all the details crucial to a diagnosis or when the patient voices an ambiguous concern.

Sample facilitations
- I understand.
- Please go on.
- I agree.
- Please continue.
- I see.

Sample probes
- And then what happened?
- What else did you notice?
- I'd like to hear more about that.

Tool 3: Laundry-list questions

Laundry-list questions give the patient a choice of alternatives in answering. Use them when you ask an open question and the patient says, "What do you mean?" For example, a patient with a toothache says, "My tooth really hurts." You respond, "What is it like?" The patient says, "I don't know what you mean," or "It just hurts!" Laundry-list questions for this common situation include: "Does the pain feel like a burn, an ache, drawing, pressure, or piercing?" and "Does the pain come on every week, every hour, every month, or every few minutes?"[13] Or you might say, "On a scale of 1 to 10, with 10 being most painful and 1 being barely noticeable, how would you rate your discomfort?" Laundry-list questions should include a wide range of possible options. Some patients hesitate to give an answer that falls outside the possibilities you suggest.

Tool 4: Clarifications

A great way to build rapport and check your understanding of patient information is to paraphrase the patient's message in your own words. For example, if a patient says, "My last dentist never told me anything before he treated me," you might respond, "So you would have been more comfortable if you knew what was going on?" If a patient says, "My gums bled and it upset me," you might clarify the message by saying, "You were worried about a possible gum problem?"

Sample clarifications
- So you mean . . .
- I hear you saying that . . .
- If I understood you accurately . . .
- Correct me if I'm wrong, but . . .

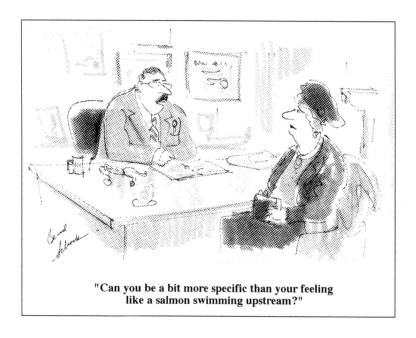

"Can you be a bit more specific than your feeling
like a salmon swimming upstream?"

Tool 5: Summaries

A brief summary of the patient's remarks reflects back to the patient what she has said. Use a summary statement to demonstrate your willingness to listen, check your understanding of the patient's message, and bridge to the next topic. A sample summary statement: "So you have pain in the tooth and in the surrounding gums, and the discomfort has been increasing during the past three or four days, is that right?"

Tool 6: Closed questions

A closed question (also called a structured or direct question) asks for a specific piece of information. It is often answered with a "yes" or "no." For example, you might ask, "Are you currently taking any prescription medications?" or "Some medical conditions affect your dental health as well as your dental treatment. Have you had any of the following?"

The advantage of a closed question is efficiency in yielding an essential piece of diagnostic information. But closed questions have two disadvantages. First, they are easily biased, skewing descriptions or prompting patients to tell you what they think you want to hear. Second, they give the patient little chance to volunteer information of potential value to your diagnosis. The following comparison of open and closed questions illustrate these disadvantages.

Closed: Is it a sharp pain?
Open: Tell me what the pain is like.

Closed: Do you eat a lot of sweets?
Open: What is your diet like on a typical day?

Closed: Does it feel comfortable?
Open: Describe how it feels.

How to Ensure the Accuracy of Patient Information

The following tips will help you clearly understand the patient's message.

Keep the answer out of your question

Leading questions, or questions that suggest a "right answer," cause patients to tell you what they think you want to hear. Closed questions are more likely to suggest a "right answer" than open questions. The following examples demonstrate how leading questions can distort patient responses.

Leading: Is the pain worse when you eat?
Not leading: What is the discomfort like when you eat?

Leading: Did you feel nausea with the medication?
Not leading: Do you have any concerns about the medication?

Leading: Did you take the medicine as directed?
Not leading: How are you taking the medication now?

Leading: You do understand, don't you?
Not leading: What questions do you have?

Keep criticism out of your questions

Avoid questions that ask patients to account for their actions or defend their behavior. Often beginning with "why," these questions are seen as negative evaluations instead of information requests. Such questions as "Why did you yell at my dental assistant?" or "How could you try to treat this yourself?" do not bring you valuable information. It's far better to say, "I don't understand this situation as much as I would like to. Please tell me how you see it."

Choose positive language

Guard against questions that scare the patient or contain emotionally charged words.[13] For example, you would ask, "Did you think it was a growth?" instead of "Did you think it was cancer?" You would say, "Tell me how the injury to your mouth occurred," instead of "Was it your fault that you got hit in the mouth?"

Deal with one issue at a time

If you try to cover multiple topics in one question, you will blur the clarity of a patient's response. For example, you will get a more accurate idea of a patient's home-care habits if you ask, "How often do you brush? How often do you floss?" instead of "Do you brush and floss every day?" You will get a clearer picture of a patient's symptoms if you ask, "What symptoms have you noticed?" instead of "Have you experienced soreness or bleeding?"

Interviewing Challenges: How to Manage the Hard-to-Talk-to Patient

Robert Frost said, "Half the world is composed of people who have something to say and can't, and the other half who have nothing to say and keep on saying it." Here are tips on managing the most common types of interviewing challenges.

The overly talkative patient

This patient responds to every question with excruciating detail or hears each question as an opportunity to say, "That reminds me of a story." The only way to protect the schedule of subsequent patients is a graceful interruption. Summarize the patient's point briefly or echo a central phrase in the patient's answer. Then, ask a more focused or specific question. Fewer open questions and more laundry-list questions will give needed structure to interviews with this type of patient. You may consider giving a suggested time limit to the interview.

The quiet patient

Although it's tempting to fire closed questions at a naturally quiet patient to force out information, persist with open questions. When silence prevails, be willing to wait for an answer instead of jumping in with another question. Nod and smile as nonverbal signs of attention. Compliment even minor contributions: "That's very perceptive. Thank you for telling me. Please go on."

The pleaser patient

A patient might try to please you by saying whatever she thinks you want to hear. With an outward appearance of complete cooperation, this patient may be responsible for as much inaccurate information as the rest of the challenging interviewees put together. Use open questions and laundry-list questions (not closed questions) with this type of patient.

The defensive patient

Closed questions are seen as more threatening than open ones. Break down defenses and build rapport by using open questions almost exclusively. Before you ask a sensitive question, explain why the information is relevant to dental or overall health.

The tired or distracted patient

Increase the animation in your voice and movement for the patient who is tired or distracted. Wait for a later visit to ask for decisions on complex treatment issues. If you must share important information, stress it carefully or put it in writing.

Interview Tool Summary

Use this approach	If you want to
Open question	Begin the interview Open a new topic for discussion Discuss a personal or potentially threatening topic
Facilitation/probe	Encourage the patient to tell you more about a topic or concern
Laundry-list question	Discover a specific piece of diagnostic information without influencing the patient's answer
Clarification	Build rapport and check your understanding of the patient's message
Summary	Check your understanding of the patient's message and bridge to a new topic
Closed question	Learn an essential diagnostic fact

Great Interview Questions

Dental goals	Dental experience	Dental condition	Treatment expectations
What are your goals for your dental health? How important is your smile to central aspects of your life, such as in your work or as a parent? What do you think your dental health will be like in five years? What do you want it to be like?	What has dentistry been like for you? What are your parents' teeth like? Tell me about your past experiences with dentistry. Has anything kept you from receiving dental treatment in the past? What was it? When was your last dental visit? What was it like? What did you have done?	What concerns (if any) do you have about your dental health? Can you eat anything you want, whenever you want? What are the positive aspects of your dental health? What are the negative aspects of your dental health? What if anything have you noticed in your mouth that suggests a need for dental treatment? On a scale of 1 to 10, how would you rate your dental health today?	What ideas do you have to improve the look and feel of your mouth? What do you most look for from a dental office?

Skill Summary

- By encouraging patients to talk, you build trust, reduce anxiety, and enhance satisfaction with your practice.

- If dental professionals do not encourage patients to tell their stories, they miss out on information central to accurate diagnoses and quality patient care.

- To become a better listener, focus on the patient's message instead of office distractions, mentally summarize the patient's remarks, pay attention to the patient's attitudes as well as diagnostic facts, and make sure your schedule allows ample time for patient conversations.

- For more effective patient interviews, listen more than you talk, refrain from interrupting, and hold writing on the chart to a minimum.

References

1. Hawes LC. A Markov analysis of interview communication. Communication Monographs 1973;40:208–219.

2. Daly MB, Hulka BS. Talking with the Doctor, 2. Journal of Communication 1975;25:148–152.

3. Korsch BM, Gozzi EK, Francis V. Gaps in doctor-patient communication: Doctor-patient interaction and patient satisfaction. Pediatrics 1968;42:855–871.

4. Levine R. The treatment conference: how to encourage case acceptance. Dental Management 1987;27:43–45.

5. DiMatteo MR, Hays RD, Prince LM. Relationship of physician's nonverbal communication skill to patient satisfaction, appointment noncompliance and physician workload. Health Psychology 1986;(5)6:581–594.

6. Beckman HB, Frankel RM, Darnley J. Soliciting the patient's complete agenda: A relationship to the distribution of concerns. Clin Res 1985;33:714.

7. Korsch BM, Negrete VF. Doctor-patient communication. Scientific American 1972;227:66–74.

8. Stewart MA, McWhinney IR, Buch CW. The doctor-patient relationship and its effect upon outcome. Journal of the Royal College of General Practitioners 1979;29:77–81.

9. Frankel R, Beckman H. Evaluating the patient's primary problem(s). In Stewart M, Roter D (eds): Communicating with Medical Patients. Newbury Park, CA: Sage Publications; 1989:86–98.

10. Nichols RG. Are You Listening? New York: McGraw-Hill; 1957:1–17.

11. Meldrum H. Interpersonal Communication in Pharmaceutical Care. New York: Haworth Press; 1994:20.

12. Geist P, Hardesty M. Reliable, silent, hysterical or assured: Physicians assess patients' cues in their medical decision making. Paper presented at the International Communication Association Convention: San Francisco; May 1989.

13. Froelich RE, Bishop FM, Dworkin SF. Communication in the Dental Office. St. Louis: Mosby; 1976:43–53.

"Do You Care?"

Starting a Successful Answer

When a patient voices a concern, there are good (and bad) ways to begin your response. This holds true whether the tough question is about insurance, treatment, or office policy. If you begin your answer well, you are more likely to reach a successful end to your conversation in less time with fewer headaches. This chapter tells how to (and how not to) begin your answers to tough patient questions.

Active Listening: A Good Beginning with Three Benefits

"The art of dealing with one's adversaries is an art no less necessary than knowing how to appreciate one's friends."

—Truman Capote

A successful start to communication is essentially "active listening," a concept first introduced by psychologist Carl Rogers.[1] It is understanding what the other person is saying and feeling, and then communicating back in your own words what you think has been said. You serve as a mirror, reflecting back to the patient the attitudes and feelings expressed. Thus, you validate the patient's position without necessarily agreeing with it.

The standard response format for acknowledgment is: You feel _____ because _____. The following examples show how the standard format can be adapted to a specific situation and to your personal communication style:

"I can certainly appreciate how you might feel (inconvenienced) because (you had to wait to see the doctor)."

"I'd probably be (frustrated) too if (I brushed and flossed every day and still had gum problems)."

"I know you are (anxious) about (how your daughter is doing during her treatment). It is (nerve-racking for a mom) to (want to help a child but not know quite what to do)."

Five Ways to Start a Patient Conversation That Ruins Your Day

Approach	Definition	Example	Disadvantage
Indifference	Showing a reluctance to communicate with the patient	A patient's question is ignored	Devalues the patient and the relationship
Insensitivity	Communicating without taking the patient's priorities into account	A patient asks, "Why haven't you joined the capitation plan offered by my union?" The dentist says, "If I joined that plan, I would have trouble covering my overhead."	Misses the opportunity to build rapport or gain patient trust
Diversion	Directing the conversation away from the patient's primary concern	A patient says, "I'd rather have a baby than go to the dentist." A staff member answers, "You have children? How nice! How many do you have?"	Postpones a patient's concern, making it more severe
Challenge	Questioning or condemning the patient's point of view	A patient who asks if insurance forms can be postdated to get coverage for treatment is told, "If I would cheat the insurance company, what makes you think I wouldn't cheat you?"	Discourages patient communication, thus endangering the patient relationship
Offense	Responding with criticism of the patient	A patient angry about an appointment delay is told, "Maybe you have to wait for us this time, but you've been late for your last two visits. I guess we're even."	Angers or insults a patient, thus damaging the relationship

If you begin a conversation by acknowledging the patient's point of view, you will receive the following benefits.

It can help you influence the patient

Fisher and Ury, authors of the well-known *Getting to Yes*,[2] state, "The ability to see the situation as the other side sees it, as difficult as it may be, is one of the most important skills a negotiator can possess. It is not enough to know that they see things differently. If you want to influence them, you also need to understand empathetically the power of their point of view and to feel the emotional force with which they believe in it."

It can lead to patient satisfaction

When patients are worried, angry, or frustrated, you want to satisfy them without giving away the store. The easiest concession is to let patients know you have considered their side. Patients do not have to get their way to feel satisfied with communication. What they need is to have their views fully heard and understood.

It can save time

If a patient voices an opinion and you respond immediately with information that contradicts that position, the patient may think, "She doesn't get it. She must not have heard what I said. I'd better say it again. Louder." And so he does. People are prone to repeat their messages until they get a clear signal that the message has been received. Ask any parent of a teenager.

> ### *Phrases to Begin an Acknowledgment of the Patient's Point of View*
>
> So you mean . . .
> I hear you saying that . . .
> If I understood you accurately . . .
> If I heard you correctly . . .
> Could it be that . . .
> Is it possible that . . .
> Correct me if I'm wrong, but . . .

Three Reasons You May Be Wrong about Paraphrasing Patients

If you already practice active listening, feel free to skip the next few paragraphs. On the other hand, if you learned the technique in dental school or dental hygiene school—and discarded it as soon as faculty stopped eavesdropping on your patient conversations—consider the following reasons you may have found it ineffective as a conversational tool.

Paraphrasing isn't for all situations

Acknowledging a patient's views by restating them in your own words is appropriate when the patient is angry, upset, scared, or confused. It is not appropriate when the patient is asking for factual information. For example, if someone stopped you on the street for directions, you wouldn't say, "I see you are feeling lost and confused in our fair city." You would simply give directions.

Imagine this exchange at your front desk:

> **Patient:** "Could I have an appointment on Friday?"
> **Receptionist:** "I perceive you as interested in a Friday appointment."

Patient: "That's what I said. I want an appointment on Friday."
Receptionist: "So if I am hearing you accurately, you desire an appointment with us on Friday?"
Patient: "Just give me the damn appointment!"
Receptionist: "I'm sensing some hostility here."

Paraphrasing isn't agreement

Once, when a patient seemed anxious about infection control, a receptionist said, "AIDS is scary, isn't it? A patient once sprayed our reception room chairs with her own disinfectant." This statement didn't bank the fires of patient fear. It added fuel to the fire instead.

Paraphrasing isn't simply repeating the patient's words

You may distrust the technique of paraphrasing because you've heard others use it and sound like a parrot. For example, if a patient says, "I simply don't want any more mercury in my system," you wouldn't respond, "So you don't want any more mercury in your system?" A stronger response would be, "Of course you don't! We are all concerned by the mercury in our food, air, and water." After acknowledging the patient's views, you might point out, "The minute amount of mercury that enters your system from an amalgam filling is flushed out of the body through natural processes. The only effect of amalgam you will experience is a health benefit—saving the structure of your tooth."

 ## The Secret to Good Paraphrasing: Voice Patient Values

What are the elements of good paraphrasing? Choose your timing with wisdom, using the technique with patients who are upset, concerned, anxious, or angry. Acknowledge the patient's views without agreeing with or adding to their concerns. Go beyond a mere repetition of a patient's words.

But the best clue for effective paraphrasing is: *Voice the value.* If you voice a patient's values in a situation, you can make a positive statement of his views. Even better, you frequently will find that you and the patient agree on the value and can search together for a way to meet it.

For example, a parent concerned about possible health problems from amalgam values safety and good health for her children. You could voice her values by saying, "Of course you want a safe filling for your daughter to protect her health. Our goal is to protect your daughter's health as well." For a patient who worries about a sore mouth after treatment, you could begin with, "That's a reasonable concern. After all, your comfort is important." If a patient says, "I just don't know about a treatment that costs that much," you could reflect his values by saying, "It is a significant investment. You deserve to know precisely what you are paying for. Perhaps it will be easier for you to make the decision if we review the benefits of having the treatment and the risks of not having it."

How to Voice the Value

Patient concern	Patient value	Example
Scheduling	Convenience, minimizing time away from work or family	"Certainly your time is important. Let's see what we can do."
Infection control	Safety from HIV transmission	"You expect safety from the transmission of disease, and I can offer you that without reservation."
Perceived treatment danger	Safety, protection of good health	"Of course you want a safe procedure that will protect your good health."
Cost	Good value, fair fee	"Everyone wants a good value for their dollar. You have a right to know precisely what you are paying for."

Dr. Jekyll Turns Mr. Hyde into a Satisfied Patient

Here are extra tips you will find valuable in managing an angry patient.

Get privacy

Invite the angry patient to a place apart from other patients. Communication is difficult if you are both playing to an audience.

Stay calm

Don't react to an emotional outburst with one of your own. One communications consultant notes, "Anger makes us overstate our case and exaggerate to get attention in the heat of the moment. We become blind to how we are contributing to the problem. Our anger should be a cue that we need to change, not attack, something. We need to talk to ourselves differently and say: 'I can't do anything about his/her behavior. I can only behave in a better way myself.'"[3]

Agree with fair criticism

You do not need to defend every aspect of yourself, your practice, and your profession. No dental office is perfect. Sometimes there is strength in admitting it. For example, if a patient says, "I hate filling out all these forms," you can agree without indicting dentistry by saying, "I know it seems tedious. Good dental care does require a lot of paperwork. We appreciate your help." You might add, "The information you provide on these forms helps us provide care that exactly meets your needs."

Ignore unfair criticism

Suppose a patient says, "There's a mistake on my bill. Don't try to cheat me!" Respond to the billing error, not the accusation. You might say, "I'm sorry! How inconvenient for you. Of course you expect an accurate statement from us. Let's see how we can fix it." You would not respond with, "I don't cheat patients!" If a patient becomes verbally abusive, however, you don't have to just stand there and take it. You can say, "I really want to resolve this, but it's hard to do so when you talk to me like that."

Ask for examples

Suppose a patient's complaint is vague, along the lines of "You people treat me like dirt." First acknowledge the complaint, "No one likes to be treated as if they aren't important." Then say, "I'd really like to know what happened. Can you give me an example of what you mean?"

Add a compliment

For example, you might glance over a patient's chart and say, "You have certainly been a good patient over the years." You might respond to a patient complaint with, "I appreciate your calling our attention to this matter. Thank you for your suggestion." When your mind is blank of any complimentary phrases, simply say, "Thanks for being so honest with me."

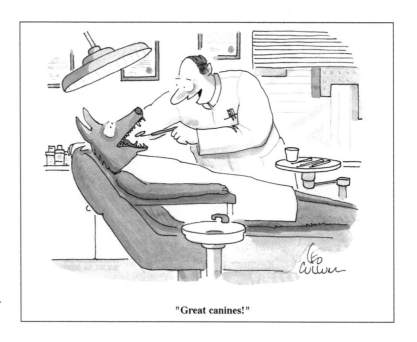

"**Great canines!**"

What not to say	What to say
We always have trouble with that.	I'm sorry! I'm sure we can straighten this out right away.
Patients complain about that all the time.	That is inconvenient, isn't it?
I don't know if there's anything I can do.	I can't make any promises, but let's see what we can do.
I don't know anything about that.	May I tell Joann about your question? She's our expert in that area.
That's not my job.	I think I understand what you need. Let me take you to Ms. Bryan.
I'll have to get back to you on that.	I'll find out about that today. May I call you tomorrow no later than 10:00 A.M.?

Skill Summary

- The ability to see a situation as the patient sees it is one of the most important skills a dental communicator can possess.

- A successful start to communication is understanding what the patient is saying and feeling, and then communicating back in your own words what you think has been said.

- If you voice the value of a patient, you not only validate the patient's point of view, but you cast a positive light on the encounter.

References

1. Rogers CR. On Becoming a Person. Boston: Houghton-Mifflin; 1961.

2. Fisher R, Ury W. Getting to Yes: Negotiating Agreement Without Giving In. New York: Penguin Books; 1981:23–25.

3. Meldrum H. Interpersonal Communication in Pharmaceutical Care. New York: Pharmaceutical Products Press of Haworth Press, Inc.; 1994:16.

"Are You Any Good?"

Building Trust in the Doctor's Skill and Judgment

"My previous dentist told me I didn't need that. Why do you say I do?" "Do you guarantee your work?" "No one ever said anything to me about gum disease. How long have I had it?" "You look too young to be a dentist." "My son is upset. What did you do to him back there?" These questions show that some patients don't give your practice the trust it truly deserves.

Patients Act on Trust More Than You Suspect

> *"It takes two to speak the truth—one to speak, and another to hear."*
>
> —Henry David Thoreau

> *"The truth would become more popular if it were not always stating ugly facts."*
>
> —Henry S. Haskins

Trust is the most important component of your patient relationships. With a mind-set of "I may not know dentistry, but I sure know people," patients use how they feel about you to determine how they feel about your message—and what they do about it. If patients trust you, they trust your message. Only after they take a measure of your character do they decide about treatment.

According to dental research, patients indicate that the honesty of their personal dentists is the most important reason they stay in a dental practice. They rate another component of trust, a dentist's knowledge of the latest techniques, as more important than gentleness, painless dentistry, or quality treatment.[1]

Patients act on trust far more often than dental professionals think they do. In a recent study by practice management consultant Suzanne Boswell, 40 percent of the dentists surveyed said patients accept treatment because they believe it is necessary. Only 8 percent of patients, however, said they accept treatment for that reason. The most important reason patients accept treatment—mentioned by 58 percent of respondents—is because they trust the dentist.[2]

Since the time of Aristotle, good communicators have recognized that if they want to be successful in reaching other people, they must be perceived as worthy of trust. If a person isn't trusted, few pay attention to the information that person offers.[3,4] One communication expert states, "We accept ideas more readily from those whom we view as authoritative and trustworthy and from those who treat us with respect and concern than from those who appear ill-informed, manipulative, or inconsiderate. Credibility affects the success of persuasion."[5] Because trust is essential to patient acceptance of your answers, all of your communication goals first require trust.

Report Card: Dentists Get High Marks on Trust

Patients trust you—especially your honesty. According to a 1991 Gallup poll, dentists are rated as the third most ethical professionals, outranked only by pharmacists and the clergy.[6] In another study, 87 percent of dentists surveyed believe that the public image of dentistry is "great" or "good."[7] Shugars and colleagues found that public respect is the most important factor influencing dentists' professional satisfaction.[8]

Five Steps to Patient Trust

The essence of trust is treating patients with integrity throughout a long-term relationship. Your image can be worse—never better—than your behavior. But what about the new patient who hasn't yet experienced your quality care? What about the patient who has been treated with great clinical skill and still seems hesitant? You need to communicate with these patients in ways specifically designed to build trust.

According to my research, patient trust in a dental professional comes in five categories:

Competence

Competence is defined as having authority, expertise, or good judgment. It means patients trust you as a clinically qualified dentist who makes accurate diagnoses and provides quality treatment.

Commitment

Commitment means patients trust your belief in the worth and "rightness" of your recommendations. When you rank high on commitment, the patient decides that you believe she really needs treatment. When you rank low on commitment, the patient suspects that you don't feel 100 percent sure of your recommendation.

Candor

Candor means patients trust you to be straight with them—tell them the whole story. It means they don't suspect you of hiding something, blocking their access to information, or leaving something out of your communication with them.

Confidence

Confidence means patients perceive you as dynamic and confident, which is usually communicated on a nonverbal level through good eye contact, an erect posture, and a strong vocal delivery. Patients respond not just to your choice of words, but how you look, sound, and move when you speak with them.

Cost fairness

Cost fairness means patients trust you to charge them an appropriate price for the care they receive. In my research with dental practices, patients voice concern about the honesty of a practice almost exclusively on issues of cost. Because financial discussions are both sensitive and complex, they require not just building trust but other communication skills as well. Chapter 6 is devoted entirely to this topic.

Faced with a patient who doesn't seem to trust the practice, you must analyze the barriers to trust for that particular patient. Which of the five categories of trust are not being met? When you have diagnosed the trust barriers, you can use an approach designed to overcome them.

If communication were easy, trust barriers would come one per patient. Unfortunately, questions from patients frequently involve more than one barrier to trust. For example, the question "Do you guarantee your work?" may reflect doubt about your competence, doubt about your commitment to treatment, or both. So, although the following communication techniques are grouped by trust category, you will often mix and match these techniques in answers to trust-related questions.

The Five C's of Trust

Trust Issues	Question Themes	Specific Topics	Sample Question
Competence	Is the dentist any good?	Diagnostic accuracy, treatment quality, consistent advice	Why do you say that? That's not what my previous dentist said.
Commitment	How personally committed is the doctor to my dental care?	Treatment guarantees, treatment need	Would you have this treatment if you were me?
Candor	Are the doctor and staff telling me everything?	Second opinions, treatment alternatives	Do you ever recommend a second opinion?
Confidence	Do the speaking styles of the dentist and staff inspire trust?	Wide variety of topics	This issue almost always remains unvoiced by patients.
Cost fairness	Is the practice trying to cheat me?	Financial policies, dental fees, insurance coverage	Why did my insurance company say you are too expensive?

What Do You Say to a Patient Who Doubts Your Competence?

Because you are a licensed professional, surpassing the requirements of extensive education and state board examinations, most patients trust your clinical abilities. But some patients do question your competence, especially when they have heard conflicting information from other sources. They make remarks such as: "That's not what I read in a magazine," or "My mother has a friend who did that and she lost all her teeth." Four communication techniques will build credibility in your clinical skill and professional judgment. The first two can be used every day to enhance patient confidence in your expertise. The last two are for use in individual conversations with doubting patients.

Highlight your professional credentials

A cab driver once told me that he had decided to join a dental HMO because he knew the dentists in the plan were the best in the area. "How do you know they are the best?" I asked. He replied, "Because every dentist in the plan is licensed by the state." Patients, even if they know little about professional standards, find comfort in official acknowledgments of dental qualifications.

The bedrock upon which your expertise rests is your education, experience, and professional qualifications. You will find practical ideas for highlighting your credentials as follows.

How to Highlight Your Credentials

- Display your diplomas on an office wall, along with the diplomas, certificates, or licenses of your entire dental team. Add other credentials such as membership certificates, completion of a residency program, and the like. Choose a prominent location and invest in fine frames.

- List your credentials—and the credentials of your dental team—in your practice brochure.

- When you or a member of your staff attend a continuing education seminar, note it in your practice newsletter. One caveat: Don't mention exotic locations. I once saw a practice newsletter with a large photo of the dentist and staff on a cruise ship, complete with funny hats and fancy drinks. Definitely not a credibility enhancer.

- When you leave for a professional conference, make sure your answering service says, "Dr. A and her dental team are attending a professional education seminar; the office will reopen Tuesday," instead of "The office is closed until Tuesday."

- When relevant to the subject, talk to patients about your professional activities. Mention what you learned by teaching at the university, speaking at the hospital, or serving on a dental society committee.

- When a team member is absent, let patients know that, "Susan is at a meeting as vice-president of the state dental assistant association," or "Maria is speaking today at the high school."

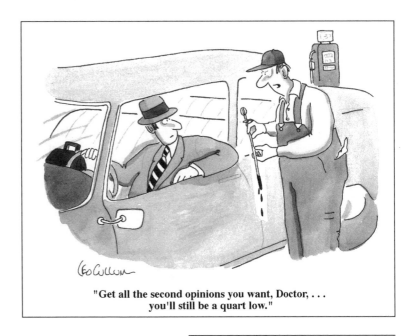

"Get all the second opinions you want, Doctor, . . .
you'll still be a quart low."

Compliment the practice in general

Naturally, you can't compliment the brilliance of your own work. But the dental assistant or hygienist can compliment the dentist's performance by saying, "He's an excellent dentist. That's one reason I like working here." The dentist can say to the dental assistant, "Thank you, that was perfect." Or the dentist can comment, "The hygienist did a superb job on your cleaning." Patients will believe and appreciate these messages of quality treatment.

Many dentists and team members are not used to emphasizing their competence; some minimize their skills in the name of professional modesty. For example, an appointment coordinator once said, "The hygienist will be right with you. She's just readying up the room a bit." This statement did not reflect the practice's careful preparation of each treatment room in accordance with universal precautions. Don't refer to your services as "just routine." Avoid such statements as: "You left me almost nothing to do!" "It's hard to go wrong with materials as fine as these." "This is one of the first procedures dental students learn." Just as patients believe messages that upgrade your service, so they will believe messages that devalue your service.

Compliment the recommended treatment in particular

Although this seems an obvious solution to doubts about clinical skill, dental professionals miss opportunities to talk about the excellence of a particular treatment recommendation for a patient's unique dental situation.

For example, if a patient says to a dental assistant, "I'm wondering if this is the best treatment for me," the dental assistant might provide a general response such as, "Well, all patients should get timely treatment." Better to say, "This is exactly the right treatment for your condition. Would you like to review the reasons it's important for your health?" Or, if a patient says to the hygienist, "I don't understand why my son has to have sealants," the hygienist should not generalize with, "Sealants are important for every child." Instead, personalize the answer with, "Sealants will be a great benefit to Jeffery. He did have those two cavities last year in spite of his enthusiastic brushing. Sealants will protect his teeth from decay."

Mention sources that the patient trusts

When patients seem to doubt your expertise, let them know you don't stand alone in your positions. A patient who seems suspicious of fluoride might be reassured to learn that fluoridation is supported by the American Dental Association, American Academy of Pediatrics, American Cancer Society, and World Health Organization. If your patient is a "Ralph Nader," you might mention that the benefits and safety of fluoridation are backed by *Consumer Reports* magazine.[9] If your patient has doubts about mercury, *Consumer Reports* also supports you on amalgam, stating that "given their solid track record and a risk that's still conjecture, amalgam fillings are still your best bet."[10] Or, you might let a patient know that your sterilization procedures meet the requirements set by OSHA and the Centers for Disease Control and Prevention.

What Do You Say to a Patient Who Wonders about Your Commitment?

Patients want to know if you really believe what you are saying or if you only partially believe what you are saying. For example, they may ask, "Would you have this treatment yourself?" The following communication approaches will let patients know you are personally committed to your professional recommendations.

Discuss your own experience

Patients will respect your personal testimony. Sample statements that use personal experience to build trust include: "I provided a similar fixed bridge for my brother-in-law. I only recommend treatment I would want for my own family." "You must make your own decision about your daughter, but I'm glad my children have the benefits of drinking fluoridated water." Or you might say, "Because I wouldn't want that treatment for myself, I wouldn't feel right about giving it to you." If you don't have personal experience to discuss, refer to your hands-on experience in treatment through case histories and specific patient examples.

Don't like this approach? As a technical person with technical training, you may prefer scientific fact to touching anecdotes. Most of your patients are exactly the opposite. They find a personal example more convincing than a research report.

Explain how you arrived at your answer

Let the patient know you are aware of a range of treatment options and have good reasons for selecting among them. Describe not only your treatment conclusion, but also the reasoning process that led to your conclusion. For example, how much treatment planning can you do while a doubtful patient watches? A patient may trust your judgment more if he sees you record the diagnosis, review his chart, study his X-rays, or write a prescription.

If you originally had the same doubts as the patient, tell how you overcame them. Suppose a patient says, "Do you really think I should use an oral irrigator? Won't it damage my gums?" You could answer: "I used to have doubts about oral irrigators too. When they first came on the market, their effectiveness varied. Not everyone got the results they wanted. But recent research shows that oral irrigators are excellent hygiene tools when used properly. Because we carefully show our patients how to use oral irrigators, we have had many patients use them with great success."

What Do You Say to a Patient Who Suspects Your Candor?

Some patients may think you are telling the truth—but aren't sure you are telling the *whole* truth. They may check to see if you are giving them a complete picture of care by asking about a second opinion. They may ask about the competency of another dentist to discover if you protect patients by being open—or if you protect colleagues in a conspiracy of silence. The following approaches will help with patients who seem to doubt the completeness of your communication.

Present a balanced message

When you are faced with a lack of patient trust, it's tempting to focus on the benefits of a proposed treatment and downplay the risks. You may be torn between your professional responsibility for full disclosure and your personal desire for persuasiveness. It's no longer a dilemma. Research shows that two-sided messages (those presenting both advantages and disadvantages) are judged as more trustworthy than one-sided messages (only advantages).[3] By giving a balanced picture of benefits and risks, you build credibility. For example, "This treatment has both benefits and risks to you. I want to be as clear as I can in describing them to help you make the decision that's right for you."

Speak at the patient's level

Research suggests that hard-to-understand language can create distrust, not lessen it.[11] Patients do not say to themselves, "Anyone who can rattle off that many big words so quickly must be really smart." Instead they think, "I didn't understand it, so I don't trust it. What's the doctor hiding under all that jargon?" Your goal is to choose words understandable to patients so they think, "This doctor speaks my language. I feel better when I know what's going on."

Open the doors to information

Nothing destroys patient trust more quickly than a perception of keeping secrets or limiting access to knowledge. Dental professionals, frustrated by a patient's reference to nondental sources of data, might say, "You read too much!" or "Where did you hear that? I wish patients would stop talking to lay people and turn to professionals for information." One irritated dentist even responded, "Your mother told you that? Where did she go to dental school?"

Patients wonder if you're hiding something when you discourage them from gathering information on their own. If a patient says, "I read somewhere that treatment doesn't work," don't waste your time quizzing them on the source ("Was it *Reader's Digest? National Enquirer?*") and then criticizing the publication ("I've never considered *Cosmo* a dental journal"). Instead, you might say, "I know there have been some articles in the press. Sounds like you've done some research into this. Would you be willing to consider additional information?" Provide brochures, research reports, and, if requested, sources for second opinions. (A patient does not have to actually read the material or get the second opinion. Your willingness to provide it is enough to build trust.)

How Can You Communicate Confidence?

When it comes to building patient trust, it's not just what you say, but how you say it. Your nonverbal behavior is as important as your word choice in communicating confidence in your abilities. Much of a patient's impression of you is based on such nonverbal aspects of your behavior as eye contact, body language, and vocal style. The following chart offers practical guidelines on developing a dynamic and confident presence.

Nonverbal Ways to Build Patient Confidence

What to try	What to avoid
Speaking with energy and appropriate emphasis	Speaking in a monotone; speaking too softly; sounding tired; using verbal fillers such as "um" or "you know"
Making direct and consistent eye contact	Looking away or down as you speak; reading the chart
Smiling as you speak; varying facial expressions	Having little change in facial expression; allowing negative reactions to show
Good posture	Slouching
Leaning forward in your chair	Leaning back in your chair
Positioning your body toward the patient	Positioning your body away from the patient
Having an open upper body position	Folding your arms
Using gestures that complement your message	Fidgeting, shuffling papers, pointing at the patient, or covering your mouth or eyes

How Should You Manage All Trust Issues?

Voice respect for the patient's concerns

When a patient expresses a concern involving any of the trust issues, begin by understanding the concern and stating it in your own words. This approach, described in depth in Chapter 2, is often overlooked on issues of trust. When someone casts doubt on your credibility, you often leap to your own defense. Two viewpoints are thrown into the conversation; you and the patient are on opposing sides. The patient will hold fast to his or her views until they are acknowledged. Simply put, you must grant credibility to gain it.

Don't say, "Trust me"

Risk communication expert Peter Sandman states, "The paradox of trust is that the more you ask people to trust you, the less they trust you."[12] Trust is built when trust is unnecessary—when patients are given a sense of control over the situation and a way to judge your abilities for themselves.

First, invite doubtful patients to judge their dental condition for themselves. For example, "That's an excellent question. Here's how you can see for yourself why I'm recommending this treatment. Hold this mirror. Do you see this—and this—in your mouth? Have you noticed X or Y symptoms? Then you have experienced for yourself the existence of this problem."

Next, involve patients in treatment decisions. Explain how your recommendation is based on the needs, wants, and preferences the patient told you about in the initial interview. If you insist on a treatment plan without input from the patient, the patient may reject it. There's nothing wrong with your plan, of course. The problem lies in the patient's suspicion of a process that excludes her. Patients are more likely to accept treatment if they are involved early on as partners in their care.

Finally, offer educational materials as a way for patients to assess your recommendations. Again, patients do not have to actually review the video or read the brochure. It's the offer that builds trust.

Questions & Answers

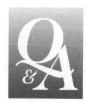

Crying Child _____

"Why is Johnny crying and his face so red? Did you have a problem?"

Possible answer   "Crying is a natural thing for children to do. Some of the procedures we do are frightening to children and they cry. Some of the work your child needed did create discomfort."

Comment   An answer plagued by unhelpful platitudes. One compliment for the dental communicator: At least he didn't try to convince the mother that her child wasn't "all that upset." (If a mother thinks her child is upset, you lose credibility by trying to convince her otherwise.) A great answer begins by validating the parent's perceptions. Then, stress your skills, compliment the child, and give the parent a sense of control over the situation.

Great answer   "Yes, Johnny's face is red. He was nervous at first, but we talked to him to help him calm down, and we were able to complete the treatment. He was a brave boy and we are proud of him. He'll feel more comfortable within the next hour or so. But here's what you can do to help him feel better in the meantime." You could add, "He did great. You might reiterate that to him when he gets home."

Best Dentist _____

"I don't know either doctor in the practice. Which one is better?"

Possible answer   "They are both excellent, highly qualified doctors."

Comment   Good start! But the answer will be more credible if it gives personal testimony and distinguishes between the two dentists based on personality, not qualifications.

Great answer   "They are both excellent, highly qualified doctors. I would be pleased to be treated by either one. Dr. A has a quieter approach; he's very reassuring, especially with anxious patients. Dr. B is more outgoing; he's great at explaining things while still being a good listener. Which would you prefer?"

Young Dentist

"You look too young to be a dentist. How old are you?"

Possible answer "I'm 28. How old are you?"

Comment Tempting as it is to try to curb patient rudeness by returning it in kind, this approach never works. Since people who ask this question are usually older than you and wish they were younger than they are, treat this question as a compliment with as much sincerity as you can muster. Throw one of your credentials into the conversation for good measure. (Giving your age is optional.)

Great answer "Why, thank you! (smile) I guess it's something I will eventually outgrow. I'm 28 and have been in full-time practice for three years since I graduated from Northwestern Dental School."

Conflicting Advice

"My neighbor (husband) (coworker) says that . . . "

Possible answer "With all due respect, Mrs. Jones, the doctor's expertise is in dentistry. She will do what is best for your dental health."

Comment This question takes many forms, touting such advice as a grandmother who calms a baby with honey on a pacifier or a neighbor who read somewhere that sealants inhibit the immune system. To answer this type of question, do not simply ask the patient to trust the experts. Instead, acknowledge the layperson's viewpoint or support the patient's right to talk about dental care with friends or family. Then present your viewpoint, stressing your years of experience with many patients.

Great answer "It's nice to have a family member encourage you. (Or: It's great to have a neighbor who is willing to discuss your treatment with you.) Dental researchers actually looked into that idea. Unfortunately, it just doesn't work. (Or: It works for very few, and unfortunately, you are one of the people for whom it won't work.) What we have found is far more successful in our experience with patients is . . ."

"Our previous dentist said that baby teeth don't hurt like adult teeth. Why should my daughter's baby teeth be fixed?"

Comment You have two goals in this answer—to win the parent's trust in your advice and to avoid criticizing the parent's relationship with a previous dentist. The following response does both by involving the parent in the development of the answer.

Great answer "It's confusing when two dentists seem to be telling you different things. I'll explain what I believe is the best way to treat Sarah. But you know your daughter best. Does she feel more, less, or the same pain as an adult? More? Well, then, you can judge for yourself the importance of keeping Sarah's mouth comfortable. Baby teeth can hurt as much as adult teeth. But teeth shouldn't hurt." (Mention the importance of baby teeth in holding space for permanent teeth, as well as the value of baby teeth in speaking, eating, and feeling confident with appearance.)

Periodontal Diagnosis _____

"My old hygienist cleaned my teeth for years and never said anything about gum disease. How long have I had it?"

Possible answer   "That's hard to say. What do you do as far as home care?"

Comment   Although this answer is an attempt to involve the patient, it sounds judgmental. It also does nothing to build trust. You need to discover what trust issue is crucial to this patient. Does she doubt the previous dentist's abilities, or does she doubt your diagnosis?

Great answer   "I can tell this diagnosis comes as a surprise. I can certainly sympathize. Were you wondering about the care at the previous office, or wondering how severe your condition is right now, or wondering when this condition began?" (Wait for answer.)

Patient wonders about the care at the previous office: "Naturally you want to know if you have had the best possible dental care. But gum disease progresses at different rates in different people—and at different rates in the same person at different stages in life. Examining your mouth now doesn't give me a clear picture of your prior periodontal health. What I can tell you is what I see today—the condition of your mouth right now based on a thorough diagnosis."

Patient wonders about the accuracy of your diagnosis: "Of course you want to know how serious your condition is. It's the only way you can decide if the treatment is right for you. If you hold this mirror, I can show you the signs of gum disease in your mouth. Then we can compare what you see in your mouth with this chart of the progression of gum disease. You will be able to determine where you are now and where you may be headed in terms of oral health."

Patient wonders when the condition began: "I can't tell you precisely how long you have had gum disease, because it progresses at different rates in different people. It can be slow or rapid, depending on such aspects of your total health as age, stress, or certain medications. We can talk about the condition of your mouth right now based on a thorough diagnosis. Then we can set up a program of treatment to bring your mouth back to the best dental health possible."

Treatment Guarantees _____

"Do you guarantee your work?"

Possible answer "There are no guarantees in life. We provide the best possible care, and the rest is up to you. We can't guarantee that you will take appropriate care of your dental work."

Comment Platitudes (or patronizing) won't work. First, find out if the patient has a particular concern about the treatment. Then, try for an answer that voices confidence in care without making promises you can't keep.

Great answer "You seem concerned about how long the crown will last, is that right? (Wait for answer.) When you are making this kind of investment, that's a reasonable question. Many of the crowns I have provided to patients have lasted a lifetime; some have not. What I can guarantee is: I will provide the right crown for your needs. I will use the finest materials. I will select an excellent dental laboratory. I will tell you everything you want to know about taking care of your new crown. But what I cannot guarantee is precisely how long the crown will last. I wish I could say I'm the most important person here, but I'm not. The difference between a crown that lasts forever and one that doesn't is the person who takes care of it a day at a time."

Treatment Recommendation _____

"Would you have this treatment if you were me?"

Possible answer "That's not a fair question because I'm not the patient! What you need to ask yourself is whether the outcome, risks, and costs are acceptable to you."

Comment First, there is no such thing as an "unfair question." (All questions are good questions.) Second, this answer misses the boat on building trust and getting action. The patient asks for a personal example—a powerful method of persuasion—but the dentist refuses.

Great answer "That's a good question. I would never recommend a treatment I wouldn't want for myself or a member of my family. In fact, my nephew had a very similar procedure, and it came out great. But this treatment is for you. Here's what you could ask yourself to be sure you are making the best decision for your particular situation: Will I be happy with the expected results? Do I understand both the benefits and risks? Am I clear on what will happen if it's done and if it isn't done? Have all my questions been answered?"

Previous Dentist _____

"When we lived on the other side of town, Dr. X was my dentist. Is he any good?"

Possible answer "Well, yes, he is. But dentists vary in skill in different dental procedures. No single dentist can be the best at everything."

Comment Oops! This answer may be honest, but it carries the potential for big trouble. Where does the conversation go from here? If asked, can you explain what the previous dentist wasn't best at? Will you explain what *you* are not best at? If you think Dr. X was a good dentist, say so. Use personal testimony to support your statements. If you are uncomfortable in supporting Dr. X, either encourage the patient to talk to Dr. X directly or let the patient know about the peer-review process in your state.

Great answer "Yes, I think Dr. X is a good dentist. I would be happy to have him as my personal dentist. In fact, I've referred patients to him when they have moved to that part of the city."

Great answer "Naturally you want to know if you have had the finest possible dental care. Dental work holds up better in some people than in others, depending on such factors as lifestyle, dental habits, or medical history. So, examining your mouth now doesn't always tell me a clear story about your prior dental care. The best person to answer your question is the doctor who provided the care. If you have any questions about your treatment, I urge you to talk to Dr. X about them. I encourage my patients to talk to me about all aspects of their care, and surely Dr. X will do the same."

If the patient presses for an evaluation of previous treatment, you might add: "It sounds to me like you are concerned about your previous dental care. Let me give you the phone number of the peer-review committee at the dental society. They help patients in situations like yours."

Second Opinion _____

"Do you ever recommend a second opinion?"

Comment Patients who ask this question seem to doubt your clinical judgment. But that's not the issue. Patients who doubt your clinical judgment don't ask about second opinions; they go out and get them. Patients who ask this question wonder about your candor—whether you are willing to open doors to patient information. (That's why they often trust you to recommend sources for second opinions.) Your answer must encourage patients to seek information from other sources, while still voicing confidence in your treatment recommendation.

Great answer   "My goal for you is to feel as comfortable with and to be as confident about this treatment plan as I am. If a second opinion will help with that, I urge you to seek one. If you have any questions about the treatment—or about the second opinion—please feel free to talk to me."

Specialist Referral _____

General practice

"You referred me to a specialist and I didn't like him at all!"

Possible answer   "We've heard that from other patients, and we no longer refer to him. If you need specialist treatment in the future, we will send you elsewhere."

Comment   This answer shows a willingness to listen to patient's preferences and adapt office policy to meet patient's needs. But it doesn't do much for your credibility—or the reputation of the specialist.

Great answer   "I am so sorry you had to visit a dentist you didn't like, no matter how excellent his skills. Let me make a note in your chart. That way, if you need future specialist treatment, we will refer you to someone with whom you will feel more comfortable."

"Do you get kickbacks from your specialty offices?"

Great answer   "What an unusual idea! (Look surprised but still pleasant.) I suppose people do wonder how we select the specialists we refer to. We refer our patients to specialists based upon the excellence of their clinical skills and patient care. The only 'kickback' we get is patients telling us they were pleased with the specialist."

Periodontal practice

"Why didn't my dentist do something before it got like this?"

Great answer   "I understand your frustration that the situation has gotten to this point. But I believe your dentist referred you at the right time. Gum disease can progress slowly and then quickly in the same person because of such factors as age, stress, or certain medications. I'm glad you acted promptly on the referral, because we will be able to save your teeth." (For additional messages, you may wish to review the answers for the periodontal diagnosis question earlier in this chapter.)

Pediatric dental practice

Possible answer "The doctors attend school two years beyond dental school to specialize in the treatment of children."

Comment This answer doesn't take full advantage of the opportunity to market your practice. In a specialty practice, additional training is not your primary selling point. Comprehensive quality service is your primary selling point. Specialty education is a supporting point to add credibility to your answer.

Great answer "Except for the toys on the floor, it looks a lot like a regular office. But actually the entire practice is dedicated to children like your Elena. Because we treat only children, we think we're better at it. The doctors not only love kids, but they have two years of education beyond dental school to treat the special needs of children. Plus, our office is designed for children, complete with a fish tank and toys. May I send you a brochure on our special approach to children?"

Skill Summary

To build patient trust in your competence

- Highlight your professional credentials
- Compliment the practice
- Compliment the treatment with messages personalized to the patient
- Cite sources respected by the patient

To communicate your personal commitment to treatment recommendations

- Discuss your own experience
- Explain how you arrived at your answer
- Tell how you overcame your doubts

To communicate an approach of candor with a patient

- Present a balanced picture (both benefits and risks) of treatment
- Speak at the patient's level and avoid jargon
- Provide educational materials
- Support those patients who seek information on their own

On all trust issues

- Acknowledge each patient's point of view
- Give patients a sense of control by sharing information about treatment

---

References

1. Kelly MA, Lange B, Dunning DG, Underhill TE. Reasons patients stay with a dentist. Journal of Dental Practice Administration 1990;7(1):9–13.

2. Boswell S. The Mystery Patient's Guide to Gaining and Retaining Patients. Tulsa: Pennwell Books; 1997.

3. O'Keefe DJ. Persuasion: Theory and Research. Newbury Park, CA: Sage; 1990.

4. Burgoon JK. The ideal source: A re-examination of source credibility measurement. Central States Speech Journal 1976;27:200–206.

5. Clark R. Persuasive Messages. New York: Harper & Row; 1984:192.

6. Hegick L, Heuber G. Pharmacists and clergy rate highest for honesty and ethics; senators and police decline. Gallup Poll News Service, May 22, 1991;54(6):1–3.

7. Gerbert B, Bernzweig J, Bleecker T, Bader J, Miyasaki C. How dentists see themselves, their profession, the public. JADA 1992;123:72–78.

8. Shugars DA, DiMatteo MR, Hays RD, Cretin S, Johnson JD. Professional satisfaction among California general dentists. J Dental Edu 1990;54:661–669.

9. Fluoridation: The cancer scare. Consumer Reports, July 1978:392–396.

10. The mercury scare. Consumer Reports, March 1986.

11. Sandman PM. Risk communication: facing public outrage. EPA Journal 1987; November: 21–22.

12. Sandman PM. Responding to Community Outrage: Strategies for Effective Risk Communication. Fairfax, VA: American Industrial Hygiene Association; 1993:42–43.

"Am I Safe?"
Reassuring Patients of Treatment Safety

"The ultimate measure of a man is not where he stands in moments of comfort but where he stands at times of challenge and controversy."

—Martin Luther King, Jr.

"How do you sterilize your instruments?" "Do you treat AIDS patients?" "Should I have my mercury fillings replaced with 'healthy' ones?" "Are my children in danger from fluoridated water?" "If X-rays are so safe, why do you leave the room when you take them?" This chapter is dedicated to the challenge of talking to patients who are afraid when you don't believe they need to be.

Communication Problem: Patients Are More Scared Than They Say They Are

Some dentists say, "My patients aren't asking about AIDS or other safety issues. It's just not a problem in my practice." If patients aren't asking, maybe it's not a problem—or maybe it's an undiscussed problem. Research shows that a sizable proportion of patients worry about dental risks, even though they don't always discuss their concerns with dental professionals.[1]

Dental risk	Patients surveyed concerned about the risk	Patients surveyed who had discussed the risk with their dentists
Contracting HIV from dental visits	30 percent	25 percent
Safety of handpieces	37 percent	15 percent
Safety of amalgam	29 percent	19 percent

Communication Analysis: Why Treatment Safety Is a Hard Sell

If patients are scared of something that actually poses little or no risk, it seems as if it should be easy to reassure them. Just tell "Mrs. Smith" it's safe, prove your point with safety statistics, and be done with it. This approach often doesn't work. Mrs. Smith distrusts your statement of safety. She disputes your statistics. She scrutinizes the research reports you give her until she finds the one study with mixed results. Why is it so difficult to convince patients of treatment safety?

Reason 1: The topics are tricky

Because you are talking about potential physical harm from the patient's perspective, the information is frightening and hard to understand by its very nature. Anxious people don't listen well. When you give patients technical information on a worrisome topic, there is often a gap between what you say and what they understand.

Reason 2: Dentists and patients disagree about dental risks

Although some patients believe the risks are high regarding amalgam, fluoride, X-rays, or HIV transmission, dentists agree with the experts that the risks are low. Risk communication is hard when the two parties disagree dramatically in their risk assessments.

Reason 3: Dentists and patients differ on communication goals

When you encounter a risk-related topic such as mercury leakage from amalgam restorations, you carefully consider scientific assessments of the risk. You think, "If only my patients knew as much about this as I do, then they would agree with me." You believe your job in talking about potential dangers is to acquire scientific knowledge and then communicate that knowledge to the patient.

Although this approach works with many patients, others do not see their safety concerns as obstacles to be overcome with expert opinion. They do not seek one-way communication, but two-way communication. They focus not just on the physical risk, but on whether they had an opportunity to contribute their views.

You see the discussion as an attempt to get your point across; the patient sees it as a sharing of information to reach a joint decision on dental treatment.

Patient Analysis: How to Diagnose a Patient's Concern about Dental Dangers

The patient who has had a bout with cancer may be more concerned than other patients about news coverage linking cancer to fluoride. A patient with MS may request the removal of amalgam fillings to relieve her symptoms. The more you know about a patient's perspective, the better you can communicate about perceived dental dangers. When a patient is worried about the safety of dental treatment, you first must diagnose the specific risk concerns of that patient. Once you diagnose the concern, you can treat it with a targeted approach to communication.

Risk Issues

Why patients may worry about risk	How you should approach their concerns
The patient's past experience creates an increased concern about a risk	Review the patient's medical/dental history; discuss her past experiences
The patient finds the risk emotionally upsetting	Take into account the public's views of risk; describe the risk as well-understood by dental professionals; endorse the patient's values; compare risks with benefits
The patient believes she personally will be affected by the risk	Choose effective risk comparisons; select safety statistics wisely
The patient has insufficient information about the risk	Provide the patient with ample information; close the gap between what he knows and what he wants to know about treatment
The patient believes he doesn't have a choice about or control over the risk	Involve the patient in treatment decisions; offer choices and alternatives
The patient isn't sure of the doctor's ability to protect patients from the risk	Incorporate trust-building techniques into your risk discussions

Risk Perception: The Dangers That Kill Are Not Always Those That Scare People

The patients who smoke, eat high-fat meals, and refuse to wear a seat belt seem to be the same patients who balk at X-rays, wonder about your sterilization techniques, and fret about the mercury in amalgam fillings. It's frustrating, especially in view of your extensive efforts to protect patient safety.

According to risk communication expert Sandman, "The risks that kill people and the risks that upset them are completely different. There are risks that upset millions of people even though they are not killing very many. And there are risks that kill millions of people without upsetting very many."[2] To successfully communicate with patients about dental risks, you must begin by understanding their risk perception.

Extensive research has analyzed the differences between expert and lay perceptions of risk.[3,4]

Experts evaluate risk as:	Likelihood × outcome
Laypeople evaluate risk as:	Likelihood × outcome × outrage factors

You and your team, as dental experts, judge the risk of HIV transmission in the dental office by considering the likelihood of transmission (essentially nil) and the outcome of transmission (eventual death from AIDS). Laypeople, however, range far beyond mortality statistics and consider "outrage factors" in their evaluation of risk.

Outrage factors are characteristics of a particular risk that influence its perceived severity.[5,6] If a dental procedure has characteristics on the less risky side, it will be seen as less worrisome and will provoke less outrage than a treatment of equal safety with characteristics on the more risky side.

Outrage Factors*

Less risky	More risky
Known	Unknown
Natural	Manmade
Ethically neutral	Unethical
Benefits	No benefits
Familiar	Unfamiliar
Voluntary	Involuntary

*Adapted from Peter M. Sandman's *Responding to Community Outrage: Strategies for Effective Risk Communication*. American Industrial Hygiene Association, 1993.

Here's an example of how outrage factors affect perceptions. According to *Science 85* magazine, the activities in the following chart all pose equal risk.[7] Each will increase your chances of dying in any year by one in a million. People don't have equal reactions to these statistically equal risks, however, because the items differ on outrage factors. For example, although 40,000 people die on U.S. highways each year, an airline crash killing 250 passengers creates more fear and outrage. People feel comfortable with the familiar, voluntary risks of car travel, yet feel anxious with the less familiar, seemingly involuntary risks of airline flights.

Increase Your Chances of Dying by One in a Million

Smoke 1.4 cigarettes
Drink one-half liter of wine
Have one chest X-ray
Fly 1,000 miles by commercial jet
Travel 150 miles by car
Ride 10 miles on a bicycle
Live for 2 days in New York
Drink Miami water for 1 year
Live within 20 miles of a nuclear power plant for 150 years

Risk Communication: How to Help Patients Make Wise Dental Decisions

The following recommendations come from applying the outrage factors to dentistry. The communication tips are not designed to force patients to accept the views of dental experts. Rather, they are designed to help you speak from a lay perspective and assist patients in making effective dental decisions.

Known vs unknown risks

The public worries when the experts do not agree. Fluoride, amalgam, and infection control have all generated controversy within the dental community. If you practice near a dentist who is opposed to amalgam fillings, you get more patient questions about the safety of amalgam. If one dentist in town opposes water fluoridation, other dentists in town who support fluoridation have a harder road to public acceptance.

Tip: When a patient seems concerned about differing opinions of experts, explain that you have examined both sides of the controversy. Give good reasons why the side you have chosen is best for your patients. Example: "Because I want to be sure the treatments I recommend are safe, I reviewed that study involving amalgam fillings in sheep. I compared it with a large number of other studies demonstrating amalgam safety. I thought about the 100 million Americans with amalgams who enjoy good health. I concluded that amalgams are safe, which is why I would choose them for my own daughter if she ever has a cavity."

Tip: Don't make negative personal remarks about your opposition. Example: "What a bunch of quacks!"

A patient concerned about X-rays said, "X-rays wouldn't be so scary if I could see something coming out of the machine." Most of the risks associated with dentistry are invisible—radiation, disease transmission, mercury leakage, fluoride content, and bacteria in water lines. Because they are invisible, they seem more unknown and therefore more dangerous.

Tip: Recognize that the invisibility of the perceived risk makes it problematic. Example: "It would be more reassuring if you could actually see bacteria being killed by the disinfectant."

Tip: Offer a related visual display as proof. Example: "What I can show you, though, is our infection control area. Would you like a tour?"

Natural vs manmade risks

People worry less about natural sources of risk, like radiation from the sun, than they do about manmade sources, like radiation from X-rays. For example, one in five people will develop skin cancer from exposure to the sun. Yet many do not worry about a picnic at the beach because the risk is perceived as "natural."

Remember the public panic in 1989 when "60 Minutes" alleged that the chemical Alar on apples put children at risk for cancer? Although the chemical was used by a small number of growers—and was removed promptly from the market—the apple industry lost over $100 million. Comparatively speaking, nature puts more dangerous chemicals in food than pesticides do.[8] But people forgive "Mother Nature" more quickly than they forgive large corporations.

Tip: Don't describe dental measures as less natural than they are. Example: "An appropriate dosage of fluoride added to water reduces tooth decay." A "dosage" sounds medicinal. Few people want something "added" to their water; it sounds unnatural.

Tip: Emphasize the natural aspects of dental treatment. Example: "Fluoride has occurred naturally in all water supplies since the beginning of time. Fluoridation simply adjusts the amount to the optimal level for dental health." Example: "A very low level of mercury is always present in the human system. It enters the body through the food we eat, the water we drink, and the air we breathe. The body naturally rids itself of mercury through the urine."[9]

Ethical vs unethical risks

If a patient's ethics or moral values are offended, the risk provokes more outrage. To illustrate, suppose a patient asks you about medical emergencies during dental treatment and you answer, "Sure, we had five last year. This year we hope to have three medical emergencies during patient treatment." Wrong answer. Your goal is to have *no* medical emergencies. The patient understands that emergencies happen. But she expects you to endorse her moral value of patient safety during treatment. As Sandman says, you do not have to reach zero medical emergencies, but you have to try.[2] A patient would not leave your practice because you had a medical emergency, but she would leave your practice if you seemed unconcerned about protecting human life.

Tip: Endorse the patient's values when you talk about risky subjects. Example: "You deserve safe dental treatment. Here's how we safeguard patients from medical emergencies, and here's how we protect patients in the event of medical complications."

Tip: Don't shrug and say, "Nobody's perfect." Tell how you strive for perfection. Example: "The goal of our community is to have a perfectly working system for the adjustment of fluoride levels in our community water supply. That's why we constantly monitor the system and consistently upgrade the equipment."

Tip: Don't compare cost with human safety or other moral issues. Examples: "Mandatory HIV testing for health professionals would be too expensive." Patients will wonder how you can put a cash value on human life. Or, "It would be cost-prohibitive to eliminate all traces of amalgam from dental office waste water." Patients will want to know why you value your checkbook more than water purity.

Benefits vs no benefits

Laypeople are talented at weighing benefits and risks. Patients recognize that different treatment options represent a trade-off in terms of esthetics, time, comfort, or cost.

Tip: Identify the risks and benefits of treatment options. For example, if a patient is concerned about the safety of amalgam, you could compare the benefits, risks, and costs of amalgam, composites, and gold fillings.

Tip: Compare the benefits and risks of treatment with the benefits and risks of no treatment. To a patient concerned about the safety of X-rays, you might say, "You are wise to consider the risk of any treatment before you make your decision. But with today's safeguards, a dental X-ray poses a far smaller risk to your health than an undetected and untreated dental problem." To a patient concerned about periodontal surgery, you might compare the possible risk of partial numbness in the tongue following the surgery to the probable risk of the loss of four teeth without the surgery.

 Risk Comparisons: Don't Say Dentistry Is Safer Than Golfing in a Thunderstorm

Hand gliding, bungee jumping, and parachuting don't seem to scare patients as much as going to the dentist does. Patients worry about the safety of dental care even though they don't worry about other activities that pose far greater risk. Is it wise to point out this discrepancy? Here are guidelines for comparisons that do—and do not—work with patients.

Don't compare apples and oranges

According to a 1992 *JAMA* article, a patient's risk of HIV infection during surgery is one-tenth the chance of being killed by lightning, one-fourth the chance of being killed by a bee sting, and one-half the chance of being hit by a falling aircraft.[10] But don't present these comparisons to patients. Because comparisons of unrelated risks ignore distinctions that patients consider important, they may damage your credibility and provoke outrage.[11]

Don't compare voluntary risks with involuntary risks

People are willing to accept higher risks in actions they perceive as voluntary, such as skiing or car racing, than in actions they perceive as involuntary, such as drinking water with pollutants or breathing secondhand smoke. The statement, "You are safer during dental treatment than you are driving to the dental office," does not reassure patients of the effectiveness of infection control procedures. Driving is voluntary; contracting HIV in a dental office is not. As Kimberly Bergalis was quoted in the *New York Times*, "I'm not asking to live in a risk-free world. I want people to be able to choose their risks. I didn't have a choice to walk out of the office and seek another dentist."[12]

Don't make comparisons with sensational events

Tempted to compare the risks of contracting HIV in your office to being struck by lightning or kidnapped by terrorists? Don't! People overestimate sensational risks and underestimate more common ones. For example, most would estimate that tornadoes and asthma cause an equal number of deaths each year. Yet tornadoes kill about 500 people a year, asthma about 3,000.[7]

Compare dentistry with other sources of the same risk[6,13]

A panoramic radiograph delivers about the same amount of radiation as three days in the sun. A bitewing examination is equal to about five days in the sun, and a full-mouth survey about nineteen days.[14] If a patient is concerned about the mercury in dental amalgam, you might say, "I certainly understand that you don't want any more mercury in your system than necessary. But as a comparison, one seafood dinner can contribute more mercury to your system than an amalgam filling."

Compare dental treatment with medical treatment

A lower GI series (barium enema) delivers 27 times more radiation to a patient that a full-mouth series of oral radiographs. A chest X-ray delivers about three times more radiation than a panoramic film.[14] Another comparison is: "A fraction of one percent of the population is allergic to mercury, but 10 percent is allergic to penicillin." Or, you can compare a dental health measure with other public health measures. Water fluoridation has been compared with various vaccine programs and with the fortification of white flour with vitamins.

Safety Statistics: Figures Don't Lie But Liars Figure

If you try to convince a patient that he personally will not be affected by a dental risk, you might tell him the chances are "one in a million." He thinks he will be that one in a million. Why aren't patients swayed by safety statistics? At first glance you might think it's because patients can't grasp numerical data. That's not it. Patients can work numbers; they do it when they buy a lottery ticket, get a car loan, or visit a casino.

Patients balk at safety statistics because they want absolute certainty. Zero risk, not minimal risk. Black and white, not shades of gray. As risk expert Donald McGregor[15] states, "We want to be removed from the natural law of chances, and we want somebody to be accountable when things go wrong."

This desire for absolute certainty makes such words as "unlikely" or "minimal risk" unacceptable to patients. Low probabilities of risk seem greater than they are.[16] In other words, if you open the door a crack to the possibility of harm, the patient mentally kicks the door wide open. How can you present facts to help patients judge the risks of dental treatment?

Choose positive language

Although a survival rate of 90 percent is equal to a mortality rate of 10 percent, people prefer positive numbers. Risk research demonstrates that people are more likely to act on information when it's presented as success rates instead of failure rates.[4] Therefore, rather than saying, "There has been no indication of any negative potential to cause harm," say, "There is every evidence of safety."

Select facts without a tie to specific numbers of people

A pollutant that will eventually cause cancer in 10,000 people sounds very serious, but one that will add less than one-tenth of one percent to the national cancer rate sounds almost negligible.[17] Statistically they are identical; perceptually they are different. Which statement would you rather hear from your surgeon: "This surgery has a 95 percent success rate," or "One thousand people had this surgery last year and only fifty of them died"? The first is a positive statistic without a connection to people. The second is a negative fact connected to individuals.

Patient Power: People Feel Safer When They're in Control

Sandman offers this risk analogy: Imagine yourself slicing a loaf of bread. Your hand is on the bread; your other hand holds the knife. Now imagine yourself holding the bread while someone else holds the knife. Your sense of danger goes way up. People feel safer when they are in control. Now imagine that someone forced you to hold the bread. The danger goes up further.[2] People are more comfortable with the risk of voluntary actions. The right to say "no" makes saying "yes" seem safer.

When you are faced with a patient who is worried about the safety of a dental procedure, it's tempting to say, "Don't worry about it. I'm the expert and I will control the situation. Sit back

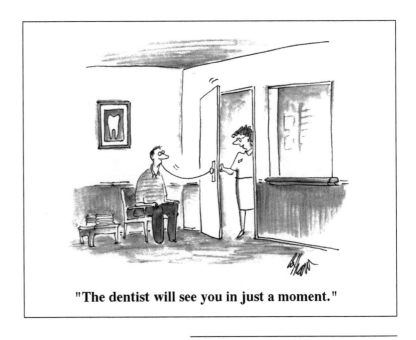

"The dentist will see you in just a moment."

and relax." For a patient worried about danger, the "sit back" and "relax" parts of the message fight each other in effectiveness. You can't keep all the control for yourself and simultaneously reassure the patient.[2]

Consider this study: Tickets to a lottery were sold for a dollar to people in an office. Participants in one group were simply handed their tickets; in another group, the participants were allowed to choose their own. Just before the drawing, ticket holders were asked to resell their tickets. The average resale price asked by those who had been handed tickets was $1.96. Those who had chosen their own tickets asked an average of $8.67. Being in control of the process apparently made people think they had a better chance of winning.[7]

If patients are partners in treatment decisions, they feel safer. How can you enhance a patient's sense of control over treatment decisions? First, the ability to listen is more important than the ability to explain. Make your treatment presentation a discussion, not a lecture. Don't talk nonstop through case presentations, pausing only at the end to ask for questions. With this approach, patients feel left out of the real action. Seek patient input before you reach your treatment conclusion. Emphasize that final treatment decisions remain always in the hands of patients.

Second, offer choices in treatment. An excellent way to enhance patient choice is to discuss treatment alternatives and the option of no treatment at all. But as the lottery study suggests, you also can offer choices that do not affect treatment outcome. For example, "We can proceed in any order with this treatment; which would you like to start with?" "Shall we begin with the right or left side?" "The top or the bottom first?" This demonstrated flexibility will increase the patient's willingness to accept needed treatment.

Have hesitations about handing over control to patients? Keep in mind that when patients are denied the chance to control their care, they may make unreasonable demands. When patients are given control, they are more likely to make reasonable requests.

Patient Information: A Risk Seems Safer if You Talk It to Death

Suppose your preschooler tells you there is a monster under her bed. What would you do? Would you tell her, "Don't be silly. There are no such things as monsters." Or would you turn on the light and look for monsters together? The second approach is more likely to lead to a quiet night of sleep for your preschooler (and for you) than the first.

Denial of risk doesn't work. Discussion of risk does. The less a patient thinks he knows about a perceived danger, the more worried he is going to be. Conversely, patients who discuss safety concerns with their dentists are less fearful and more likely to accept dental care.[1] Providing information not only reduces patient anxiety and encourages treatment, but it creates an image of clinical competence for a dental practice.[18]

By talking to patients about real or perceived dental dangers, you inoculate your patients against anxiety. Try the following communication techniques:

- Explain universal precautions as a matter of course and offer an infection control tour to new patients.
- Get brochures on risky issues—fluoride, X-rays, amalgam, infection control. Leave them out in plain view; don't make patients ask for them.
- When an issue is "hot," write a letter about it to your patients. Leave copies at the front desk for patients to peruse and take home.
- Buy your dental team buttons that say, "We welcome your questions."

Patient Confidence: First They Trust You, Then They Trust Your Message

Whether the issue is amalgam, fluoride, infection control, X-rays, or anesthesia, patients must trust you before they trust your message. From the trust-building techniques in Chapter 3, those best suited to safety discussions are included in the following chart.

Applying Trust Techniques to Safety Issues

Trust technique	Example
Compliment the practice in general	"When I first started working here, I was reassured by how seriously the doctor takes every safety precaution."
Compliment the treatment in particular	"I just wanted you to know that the doctor reviewed your medical history carefully and has planned today's treatment in view of your diabetes condition."
Mention sources the patient trusts	"We meet—and at times exceed—every infection control guideline recommended by the Centers for Disease Control and Prevention."
Give personal testimony	"I have amalgam fillings in my own mouth." "My mother comes here. I use the same infection control procedures for you as I do for her."
Tell how you came to your decision on the issue	"I wanted to make sure that every child in the practice (yours and mine included) was safe in terms of fluoride. After reviewing more than 100 studies, I came to the conclusion that fluoride treatments are not only safe for children's health, but essential for preventing tooth decay."
Speak at the patient's level	"Trying to diagnose without X-rays is like trying to do an exam with the lights off. I can't see everything necessary to get a complete picture of your dental health."
Open doors to information	"That's an excellent question about sterilizing instruments. May I give you a tour of our infection control area? And here's a brochure to take home."
Show respect for the patient's point of view	"Of course you want to make sure the treatment is safe, not just for now, but in the long run."

Questions & Answers

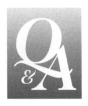

AIDS and Infection Control _____

"Do you treat AIDS patients?"

Possible answer   "Yes, but we treat them after regular hours when all of our normal patients have gone home."

Comment   The first problem with this answer is casting AIDS patients as not "normal." The second is casting doubt on infection control procedures. Patients are reassured to hear that you use the same precautions with all patients, regardless of HIV/AIDS status.

Possible answer   "Yes. We are required to by law."

Comment   This answer cheats you of credibility. You treat AIDS patients because you are dedicated to access to dental care for all citizens. Also, the answer bypasses the patient's concern regarding safety of dental treatment.

Great answer   "We assume that we do. That's why we have a strict adherence to universal precautions with every patient. (You might smile and add: Even my mom.) May I give you a tour and show you what we do to protect patients?"

"Have you been tested for AIDS?"

Possible answer   "Yes." (Wait for patients to ask the results of the test.)

Comment   Although the question is intrusive, choose a response that opens the door to a conversation about the effectiveness of your infection control procedures.

Great answer   "Yes, I was tested as part of my life insurance policy. The results were negative."

Comment   You may hesitate about this answer because negative results on an AIDS test don't guarantee patient safety from disease transmission. On the other hand, it's the answer many patients want to hear. If you are comfortable with the answer, use it and then follow up with information about universal precautions.

Great answer   "We take patient safety very seriously here. The best reassurance of safety is following infection control procedures. Because we have so much faith in our universal precautions, we know you are safe. Let me show you what we do in terms of infection control."

(The hygienist brings in instruments in a sealed package.) *"Do you throw those instruments away after each patient?"*

Possible answer "Of course not. Do you know how expensive that would make your dental care?"

Comment Do not compare safety with cost. It sounds as if you value money more than people.

Great answer "That's a good question. Every item used in your treatment is either sterilized or brand new. The instruments in this bag are sterilized for your protection. If an item can't be sterilized, it is disposable and thrown away after each patient."

"Do you sterilize your handpieces?"

Great answer "Certainly. It's an important part of our infection control program designed to keep you safe in the dental practice. Would you like to see what else we do?" (Note: When a patient is scared, verbal reassurance may not be enough. That's why many of these answers include an offer of an infection control tour.)

"How is AIDS most likely to be transmitted in the dental office?"

Possible answer "Through invasive procedures, especially those that involve bleeding."

Comment Name one dental procedure that certain patients wouldn't find "invasive." You haven't eliminated any areas of perceived risk with this answer.

Possible answer "The most dangerous procedure in the dental chair would be unprotected sex. But we don't get a lot of that here."

Comment Patient safety is a poor topic for humor. Display your wit on other matters.

Possible answer "In terms of your safety, consider these statistics: Your chances of dying from general anesthesia are 1 in 10,000. Your chances of dying from penicillin are 1 in 100,000. Your chances of contracting AIDS from an HIV-positive dentist are 1 in 250 million. So you see, your chance of contracting AIDS in the dental office is minimal."[19]

Comment Avoid the use of negative statistics. Patients focus more on the "one" than on the second number, whatever it is. These statements translate into, "So it's possible to get AIDS here."

Great answer "It isn't. Infection control procedures protect patients from the transmission of disease. After the Acer case, the Centers for Disease Control studied nearly 32,000 patients treated by HIV-infected health-care workers. They did not find a single case of HIV transmission through medical or dental treatment.[19] I'll be happy to show you exactly what we do. And you know, I treat my own family here. I follow the same precautions for you as I do for them."

"What should a patient do if her dentist doesn't wear gloves?"

Great answer   "If you know someone who has a concern about infection control, encourage her to sit down and talk to the doctor about it. I'm sure the dentist will be happy to reassure her. And if she isn't reassured, then she should think about finding another dentist."

Amalgam

"With all the controversy over mercury fillings, do you think they are safe?"

Great answer   "I do. I have them in my own mouth. Research clearly points to amalgam safety. Plus, dentists have an amazing track record on amalgam with 100 million patients over a century and a half. That's why I chose amalgam fillings for my own children."

"I read somewhere that the mercury in dental fillings can leak out and enter the body. Is that true?"

Great answer   "Almost all of the mercury in a filling is locked in as it hardens. As an analogy, you put eggs in a cake, but once the cake is baked, you can't get the eggs out. (Or, as an analogy, you put pigment in paint to change the color, but after you paint a room, you can't take the pigment out.) The tiny amount of mercury that may leak out of a filling is flushed out of the body through natural processes. And in comparison, it is a far smaller amount than we get from our food, air, and water.

"I have had terrible headaches. Could they be caused by the mercury in my fillings?"

Possible answer   "It's highly doubtful. An allergic reaction to dental amalgam is extremely rare."

Comment   Although an accurate answer, this answer ignores the patient's total health needs.

Great answer   "Those headaches must be very uncomfortable. Based upon your health history and dental examination, your headaches are caused by something other than your fillings. We will do all we can to help you find the cause of your headaches, perhaps by giving you a referral to a fine physician if you don't have a personal doctor."

"Maybe I should have my fillings removed to cure my arthritis. What would the dental scientists say about that?"

Possible answer   "There is no valid data to demonstrate clinical harm to patients from amalgam fillings. Nor is there sufficient evidence that having them removed will prevent adverse health effects."

Comment   Such language! It's both clinical and negative.

Great answer   "The dental scientists would say that removing your fillings in the hopes of curing your arthritis would be unfair to you because, unfortunately, it just won't work. I would be happy to share information with you from such reputable sources as the U.S. Public Health Service and the National Institute of Dental Research that clearly supports the safety of amalgam fillings. Would you be willing to talk with your personal physician about relief from your symptoms? I know how painful arthritis can be."

Fluoride

"I don't want my child to have fluoride treatments. I read somewhere that fluoride is poisonous."

Possible answer   "In large quantities fluoride can be a poison, as can many other products. But if it is taken in the recommended dosage, it has been proven to help strengthen the teeth and help prevent cavities."

Comment   This answer is not particularly reassuring. Some parents could translate it into: "So fluoride is poison, but you use it anyway."

Great answer   "You are wise to be cautious and ask questions about every treatment for your child. What about the risks of fluoride treatments? I reviewed the hundreds of studies on fluoride very carefully, and based on the research and my personal experience with children over the years, fluoride treatments are safe if done properly—which we definitely do. I wouldn't want my children to go without them; fluoride strengthens the teeth and prevents cavities. It is key to keeping your daughter cavity free."

"I read somewhere that fluoride can cause cancer. So I drink bottled water."

Great answer   "Certainly you should drink whatever makes you most comfortable. But would you be interested in more information? Great. Some of the world's leading medical organizations—including the National Cancer Institute—have conducted exhaustive research into any possible link between water fluoridation and cancer. There isn't one. The main health effect of fluoride in water is protecting teeth from decay." You might add: "Did you know that fluoride occurs naturally in all water everywhere? Fluoridation is adjusting the amount of fluoride in water. In our town it means putting in some fluoride; in other towns it means taking some out."

Water Lines _____

"I read in the newspaper that germs build up in the water lines of dental offices and spread disease between patients. Is that true?"

Great answer "Certainly you want to make sure that the water—or anything else that goes in your mouth—will keep you healthy. Let me show you what we do as recommended by the Centers for Disease Control and Prevention. We flush the water like this every morning and again between every patient." (Demonstrate flushing the dental-unit water lines.)

X-Rays _____

"Do I really need X-rays?"

Great answer "Yes, you do. I recommend X-rays only when they will show something important about your dental health that I can't see with just my eyes. In your case, we need the X-rays to check for small cavities between the teeth. If we catch the cavities early, we will keep down your dental costs as well as protect your health. Let's look at your X-rays together so you can see for yourself what they show."

"I don't want any X-rays. I think they're dangerous."

Possible answer "That could be considered negligent dentistry. I won't provide that type of care and a patient shouldn't consent to it."

Comment Like killing a fly with an Uzi. Try other approaches first. Then if you need a "big gun" answer, present it as, "Because I believe so strongly that X-rays are essential to the diagnosis of such life-threatening conditions as oral cancer, I simply cannot proceed without them. To do so would be a great disservice to your health."

Great answer "You want to be sure you are protecting your health? This X-ray, giving about the same amount of radiation as five days in the sun, poses a far smaller risk to your health than an undetected and untreated dental problem. An X-ray is essential to the diagnosis of not just cavities but other serious health conditions, such as bone infections and tumors." You might add: "Inspectors from the state Office of Radiation Safety come into our office regularly and monitor our X-ray equipment to be sure it is safe and effective. Let me show you the letter we received from them this year."

*"If X-rays are so safe,
why does your girl leave
the room?"*

Possible answer   "Because the button is outside the door."

Comment   Tempting! But patients with a modicum of scientific literacy need much more. Another "wish I could but shouldn't" answer is, "Give her that leather apron you're wearing and she'll stay."

Possible answer   "She's not my girl! Anyway, as I'm sure you recognize, there is a big difference between getting X-rays every couple years and being exposed to radiation on a daily basis. I would never ask my professional staff to place themselves at risk."

Comment   First, be a role model, not a nag. Instead of correcting a patient's language, simply persist with professional titles for your team. Second, try comparing benefits as well as risks.

Great answer   "That's a good question. My professional staff take about 400 X-ray films each week, compared with one set of X-rays every two years for the typical patient. As another comparison, patients receive an important benefit from X-rays that my staff doesn't—the early diagnosis of dental problems."

*"How much radiation is my
child being exposed to?"*

Possible answer   "I don't know how much radiation is being absorbed. I can only give you the amount that is coming out of the machine. It is a minimal amount. We do try to reduce your child's exposure by using a lead apron with a thyroid collar and high-speed film."

Comment   Don't begin your answer with an "I don't know," especially to make a distinction irrelevant for most parents. Also, you don't "try" to reduce exposure; you do reduce exposure.

Great answer   "The amount is comparable to about three days of sunlight. You want to be sure X-rays are safe for your child, and here's how we keep your child's exposure to a minimum. First, we use the latest in X-ray equipment, high-speed film, and a lead apron with a thyroid collar. Second, we take only necessary X-rays to detect conditions potentially dangerous to your child's health. I give X-rays to my own child to detect dental problems I otherwise couldn't see."

Prescription Medication _____

"Is this prescription safe?"

Great answer "Naturally you want to be sure this medicine is safe for your particular health situation. The scientific literature shows it is as safe as any powerful prescription medication can be. You may experience the minor side effects of (drowsiness, an upset stomach), but those will disappear when you finish the prescription. So that you are fully informed in your decision, you should know that the drug has been associated with isolated instances of (heart problems, increased blood pressure) especially in older patients. But more than 99 percent of the millions of people who have taken this medicine over the years have had no side effects whatsoever."

Sealants _____

"I read in the paper that sealants release estrogen-like chemicals that can cause cancer or reproductive problems. How could you recommend them for my son?"

Great answer "You are looking to protect your son's health, and you are wise to ask questions about any treatment for your child. I carefully reviewed that study on sealants (conducted not on people but on cell cultures in a laboratory) along with a number of other studies on sealants. We know that some chemicals leak out of sealants. This occurs almost entirely right after the sealants are put in. Almost all of these chemicals dissolve and are flushed out of the body in about a day. So, your child's contact with the chemicals is very, very limited. I believe sealants are safe. I want my children to have them, especially in view of the benefits. But he is your son, and we will go with whatever decision makes you most comfortable."

Skill
Summary

- In discussions about dental dangers, patients seek two-way (not one-way) communication with you. They focus not just on the physical risk, but on whether they had an opportunity to contribute their views and participate in decisions about dental treatment.

- Communication methods to help patients recognize the safety of dental treatment:

  - Explain how the treatment is well understood by dentists and dental researchers

  - Emphasize the natural aspects of the treatment

  - Compare the benefits and risks of the recommended treatment, alternate treatments, and no treatment

- Do not compare dental risks with unrelated risks (such as driving to the dental office) or sensational events (such as being eaten by a shark). Because these comparisons ignore distinctions that patients consider important, they may damage your credibility. Instead, compare dental risks with other sources of the same risk or with other medical treatments.

- Patients prefer positive numbers. Do not use negative statistics connected to individuals: "The failure rate is one in 10,000." Instead, use positive statistics without a connection to people: "The success rate is 99.99 percent."

- When patients have a sense of control over their dental treatment, they feel safer. Involve all patients in treatment decisions and offer choices or alternatives when possible.

- Denial of risk doesn't work. Discussion of risk does. By talking to patients about real or perceived dental dangers, you inoculate your patients against anxiety.

References

1. Gerbert B, Bleecker T, Saub E. Risk perception and risk communication: Benefits of dentist-patient discussions. JADA 1995;126:333–339.

2. Sandman PM. Responding to Community Outrage: Strategies for Effective Risk Communication. Fairfax, VA: American Industrial Hygiene Association; 1993.

3. Covello VT, Slovic P, Von Winterfeldt D. Risk Communication: A Review of the Literature. Washington, DC: US Environmental Protection Agency, Office of Policy Analysis; 1987.

4. Fischhoff B. Risk: A guide to controversy. In National Research Council: Improving Risk Communication. Washington, DC: National Academy Press; 1989:211–319.

5. Fischhoff B, Lichtenstein S, Slovic P, Derby SL, Keeney R. Acceptable Risk. Cambridge: Cambridge University Press; 1981.

6. Covello VT, Sandman PM, Slovic P. Risk Communication, Risk Statistics, and Risk Comparisons: A Manual for Plant Managers. Washington, DC: Chemical Manufacturers Association; 1988.

7. Allman W. Staying alive in the 20th century. Science 1985;October:31–41.

8. Ames BN, Magaw R, Gold LS. Ranking possible carcinogenic hazards. Science 1987;236:271–280.

9. When your patients ask about dental amalgam. JADA 1991;122:81.

10. Daniels N. HIV-infected professionals, patient rights, and the "switching dilemma." JAMA 1992;267:1368–1371.

11. Covello VT, Allen FW. Seven Cardinal Rules of Risk Communication. Washington, DC: U.S. Environmental Protection Agency, Office of Policy Analysis; 1988.

12. New York Times; February 9, 1991: A1.

13. Covello, VT. Risk communication: An emerging area of health communication research. In SA Deetz (ed): Communication Yearbook 15. Newbury Park, CA: Sage Publications; 1992:359–373.

14. Frederiksen NL. X-rays: What is the risk? Texas Dental Journal 1995;February:68–70.

15. Ecenbarger W. The home of the not so brave. Chicago Tribune Magazine; July 30, 1992:18–21.

16. Slovic P, Fischhoff B, Lichtenstein S. Rating the risk. In Glickman TS, Gough M (eds): Readings in Risk. Washington, DC: Resources for the Future; 1990:62–75.

17. Sandman PM. Risk communication: facing public outrage. EPA Journal 1987; November: 21–22.

18. Hamilton MA, Rouse RA, Rouse J. Dentist communication and patient utilization of dental services: Anxiety inhibition and competence enhancement effects. Health Communication 1994;6:137–158.

19. Siew C, Chang SB, Gruninger SE, Verrusio AC, Neidle EA. Self-reported percutaneous injuries in dentists: Implications for HBV, HIV transmission risk. JADA 1992;123:37–44.

"Is It Worth It?"

Motivating Patients to Accept Treatment

"If you want to persuade people, show the immediate value and relevance of what you're saying in terms of meeting their needs and desires."

—Herb Cohen

"I detest life insurance agents. They always try to convince me that someday I will die, which is not so."

—Carl Sandburg

"Why do I need treatment if nothing hurts?" "What will happen if I do nothing?" "Why will it take so many visits?" "I just want this tooth filled; don't try to talk me into anything else." "What if I just have all my teeth pulled like my parents did?" "I don't have time for treatment right now."

Although you wish patients would just say "Yes, Doctor," when you make a case presentation, some patients don't accept treatment. If your case acceptance rate is above 70 percent, you are ahead of the game. On the average, four of ten patients fail to do what their doctors recommend.[1]

Why do some patients say "no" to treatment? Is it because they don't understand the dental information? Do they miss the seriousness of their conditions? Is it because they don't feel capable of following treatment plans? Are they busy, lazy, forgetful? Is it all of the above? This chapter takes a close look at the barriers to treatment acceptance and offers practical solutions for bringing patients to "yes" in case presentations.

Case Acceptance Brings Patient Benefits Plus Practice Success

Without a doubt, treatment acceptance is good for patients. When patients follow through on your recommendations, they can eat better, talk better, smile better. Treatment even saves lives. Simultaneously, case acceptance is good for your practice. When patients assent to treatment, a practice is productive and profitable. Quality dentistry exists only when patients agree to it.

A Persuasive Plan: Five Steps to Patients Saying "Yes"

When patients hear your treatment recommendations, they carefully evaluate your messages to decide whether to do what you suggest. Here are five issues in patient acceptance of treatment.

Step 1: Understanding

Research shows that patients fully understand what their doctors tell them only 15 percent of the time. Further, although 90 percent of patients value having as much information as possible from their doctors, the information they desire often is not provided.[2] The first step in persuasion is closing the gap between what the patient knows and what the patient wants or needs to know.

Step 2: Need

Patients listen to your explanations of dental conditions and ask themselves: "Is my dental health really threatened?" "How bad is it?" "Must I take care of it right away or can it wait?" It's a rare patient who accepts a treatment plan simply to defer to a doctor's orders. Instead, patients decide for themselves about the severity of their dental conditions. If they judge their dental problems to be serious and immediate, they are more likely to listen to your treatment recommendations.

Step 3: Value

Patients next consider if treatment is worth their time, inconvenience, and money. In deciding whether to do what you suggest (or do something else or do nothing) patients will select the action with the greatest benefits and the smallest disadvantages. To gain patient agreement, you must maximize the benefits and minimize the disadvantages of treatment from the patient's point of view.

Step 4: Identity

Some patients don't accept treatment because they don't believe they are capable of doing it. For example, a patient may see himself as too busy (or disorganized) to schedule the necessary appointments. Other patients don't see themselves as the kind of people who deserve excellent dental care. A patient may say to herself, "A crown probably is ideal for a lot of people, just not for me." A most effective but seldom used approach to persuasion is assisting patients in identifying themselves as the type of people who are capable of following through on treatment.

Step 5: Action

Believing isn't doing. For example, you value your children's education, but somehow you've missed the last three PTA meetings. You believe in protecting the environment, but your to-be-recycled newspapers are still stacked in the garage. Similarly, some patients recognize the seriousness of their dental conditions, agree with the benefits of prompt treatment, perceive themselves as responsible dental patients, but still don't take action. How do you get those patients in the chair? How do you keep them motivated in home care? Specific techniques in persuasion will help increase patient compliance with necessary treatment.

Five Steps to Persuasion

Issues	Definitions	Examples
Understanding	Patient finds dental information inadequate, confusing, or hard to believe	"I don't understand why you fill baby teeth when they fall out anyway."
Need	Patient isn't sure of the existence, severity, or immediacy of a dental problem	"How long can I put this off?" "Since it doesn't hurt, why do I need anything done?"
Identity	Patient doesn't consider herself the type of person who invests in care	"I just don't know if this treatment is for me. I figured I'd lose my teeth like my dad did."
Value	Patient isn't sure the treatment is worth the time or inconvenience	"I don't have time for this right now." "Why does it take so many visits?"
Action	Patient doesn't comply with treatment or home-care instructions	"I forgot about my appointment." "I don't have time to floss."

Understanding: How to Be Clear When It's Confusing

Explaining dental care to patients is not easy. The information is unfamiliar, the language difficult, the concepts hard to picture. Complicating your task is the low level of functional literacy for many Americans. According to the Educational Testing Services in Princeton, one-quarter of U.S. adults cannot read a job application, determine the difference in price between two items, find a designated intersection on a street map, or enter background information on a simple form.[3]

Many patients in our health-care system are dangerously confused. In fact, 50 percent of patients leave their doctors' offices not knowing what they are supposed to do to take care of themselves.[2] More than 30 percent of patients who receive prescriptions use their medication in ways that could pose serious threats to their health.[4]

How Much Do Your Patients Know about Dental Treatment?

According to a 1995 consumer research project from the Massachusetts Dental Society,[5] 77 percent of patients think their dentist keeps them informed about new techniques. However:

- 21% are unfamiliar with caps, crowns, and root canals
- 33% are unfamiliar with gum treatments and bridges
- 42% are unfamiliar with such cosmetic procedures as bonding and veneers
- 50% are unfamiliar with bleaching, whitening, or dental implants
- 33% did not know that children get fewer cavities today than their parents did

As shown by the table above, dental patients consider themselves "well informed." Yet many are unfamiliar with treatment procedures central to quality dentistry. This is not just an educational challenge, it is a marketing opportunity. For example, four in ten patients are unfamiliar with bonding and veneers. The enterprising dental communicator who informs them about cosmetic dentistry could promote patient knowledge as well as practice growth. Here are communication techniques to help create a clearer understanding of dental care.

Know the patient

The better you know your patients, the more accurately you can match your message to their backgrounds, knowledge, and interests.

Make the message complete

Researchers have found that in a typical 20-minute medical visit, physicians spend less than one minute giving patient information.[6] Most patients want more information than they get. They especially want to hear about the treatment, the use of equipment, and how patients are expected to act. Further, patients are nearly unanimous in their dislike of dentists who start treatment without explanation.[7]

Focus on your main message

On the other hand, patients do not want a word-for-word rendition of the last clinical seminar you attended. If you know your communication goal, you will be more likely to stick to your topic and tell just the important facts rather than wandering off on a related-but-irrelevant point. By focusing on specific messages, you can save time—and keep the patient's attention.

Start strong

People tend to remember the first and last things you say and to forget the middle of your message. Put your most important statements first and last for long-term impact.

Give the big picture

A preview statement will help patients create an outline or mental model of your explanation. For example, "There are four phases to your treatment plan," or "First let's discuss your dental condition, then talk about the treatment itself."

Use short sentences

Brief statements containing one idea are easier to understand than long, complex statements containing several ideas.

Use familiar words

Your goal is to have patients understand your message so well that they can repeat it later when family members ask, "So what did the doctor say?" Simple, familiar words will make your message memorable as well as understandable. Many patients will not ask for an explanation of a clinical term. They will create a distorted lay translation of your message rather than risk the embarrassment of appearing uninformed.

Highlight key points

Use your delivery style to make important messages stand out. (You want key points to be in **boldface**.) Pause before and after crucial messages. State them slowly and forcefully, then resume a more relaxed style for background information.

Use examples

Examples make your explanation specific, interesting, and memorable. If you tell a story, you can demonstrate the effect of your information on the life and health of the patient.

Don't do all the talking

People remember 20 percent of what they hear and 90 percent of what they themselves say, according to a study by the U.S. Department of Health and Human Services. So, if you let patients explain, they will remember more.

Statements to Involve Patients in Treatment Explanations

How would you describe the dental problem?

What (if any) experience have you had with this in the past?

What do you think is causing the problem?

What do you think will help clear up this condition?

Just to make sure I didn't leave anything out, would you mind telling me how you are going to take this medication?

To make sure I've been clear, give me a quick summary of your home-care plans.

Words to Leave Out of Treatment Explanations[8]

Word type	Description	Examples
Relative words	Because these words get their meaning through comparisons, they may mean something different to patients than to you	Smaller, more, longer, frequently, sooner, in a while
Secret antagonizers	These words may be perceived as condescending	Using "he" to refer to both men and women; calling a Cynthia "Cindy" or a Richard "Dick"; calling a patient "son" when you are not his parent
Scary words	Words that can create anxiety for patients	Cut, drill, needle, extraction
Jargon	Words that hold meaning only within a particular area of expertise	Amalgam restoration instead of silver filling; fermentable carbohydrate instead of starchy food

Understanding: How to Be Convincing When It's Hard to Believe

Some dental messages are difficult to understand not because they include unfamiliar words or complex concepts, but because they run counter to intuition.[9] Certain dental ideas conflict with patients' deeply held theories about how health care or the world works. This conflict can lead patients to reject or misunderstand fundamental aspects of preventive dentistry.

Following are examples of dental messages that are hard to believe because they conflict with common-sense notions:

Dental message: In spite of a lack of symptoms, you have a potentially serious periodontal problem.
Common-sense notion: I can't have a serious dental problem because I'm not in any pain.

Dental message: A little bleeding when you floss is normal; please floss every day.
Common-sense notion: If my gums bleed when I floss, I must be damaging my mouth. I'd better stop doing it.

Dental message: That cavity in your son's baby tooth should be taken care of.
Common-sense notion: Why fix baby teeth when they fall out anyway?

Dental message: Choose a soft-bristled toothbrush.
Common-sense notion: Stiff bristles should clean better than soft ones.

When a patient holds an erroneous (but plausible) belief about dentistry, should you jump in with expert information proving him wrong? No. This approach communicates an underlying message of "Anything that I think of off the top of my head is better than what you have thought of, even if you have been thinking about it a long time." The patient may respond by ignoring, denying, or disbelieving your message. Instead, you must validate the patient's point of view, then create an explanation that makes sense in the patient's world.

Suppose you tell a patient he has a serious problem in his mouth due to periodontal disease. He finds your message hard to believe because he has no symptoms. Purdue professor Katherine Rowan recommends the following approach[9]:

Explaining a Message That's Hard to Believe

Technique	Application
Restate the patient's erroneous but plausible notion and acknowledge its plausibility	"It's hard for any of us to understand that a physical problem exists when we don't have any symptoms. After all, when you sprain an ankle or have a cold, you are uncomfortable."
Demonstrate the inadequacy of the patient's belief by comparing it with other ideas familiar to the patient	"Periodontal disease is similar to medical conditions like high blood pressure or anemia that can be present without the person's knowledge and can become serious without any outward symptoms."
Demonstrate the greater adequacy of your dental concept	"Would you like to see how gum infections can progress to an advanced stage even though the mouth looks normal? Let's take a look at this chart . . ."

Need: How to Overcome the "It Ain't Broke, Don't Fix It" Attitude

You and the patient must agree on the nature of the dental problem before you can agree on a treatment plan. For example, if a parent thinks a cavity a year is normal for children, she won't be motivated to make changes in her child's diet and home-care habits. If a patient is not convinced of the need for treatment during a discussion of her dental condition, she cannot be convinced to take action.

Insight on how to convince patients of the need for dental treatment comes from communication professor Kim Witte.[10,11] Summarizing decades of research on persuasion, she argues that when individuals are informed of a threat to their health (like a dental problem) they appraise the seriousness and likelihood of the danger. If the danger is perceived as irrelevant or insignificant, there is no motivation to process the message further. The potential for patient action stops.

If patients believe themselves to be threatened by serious harm, they are motivated to begin a second appraisal, which is an evaluation of the effectiveness of the recommended action to deal with the threat. If patients believe they can successfully avert the threat to their health, they are motivated toward danger control. They seek strategies to protect themselves and are likely to adopt a treatment plan.

If, however, patients believe they cannot prevent the threat, they are motivated toward fear control. They seek ways to deal with the fear, not with the danger. They may deny the threat, ignore the message, or lash out at you as the bearer of the news.

How Patients Deal with Health Threats

Step One: Appraising the Problem	
If patients believe the threat is minimal or irrelevant:	Patients stop listening to the message
If patients believe the threat is serious and likely:	Patients continue to listen and move to Step Two
Step Two: Appraising the Solution	
If patients believe they are capable of taking effective action to avert the danger:	Patients will adopt the recommended action, such as accepting a treatment plan
If patients believe they are incapable of taking action or believe the action will be ineffective:	Patients will engage in fear control processes such as denial, avoidance, or hostility

As an example, suppose you have a patient who is at risk of oral cancer because of his use of smokeless tobacco. If he perceives his situation as low threat, he would say to himself, "It's not like I'm smoking. A chew once in a while isn't going to hurt me."

If he perceives his situation as high threat/high effectiveness, he would say to himself, "I'm at risk of oral cancer from chewing tobacco. I don't really want to quit, but I can and will."

If he perceives his situation as high threat/low effectiveness, he would say to himself, "I'm at risk of oral cancer, but there's nothing I can do. I can't quit. I'm too old to change. That dentist should keep his nose out of my personal business."

To follow Witte's advice in convincing patients of the need for treatment, your first step is to convince patients of the seriousness of their dental condition. The following points explain how to do that. Your second step is to outline specific steps to cure the dental condition, emphasize the effectiveness of the recommended treatment, and convince patients they are capable of taking action. The next section (Identity) will assist you with this second step.

Prove the existence of the dental condition

Patients will accept your recommendations only if they believe they actually have the dental problem. Consider this example: Citizens in Thompson Canyon, Colorado, were warned of a flood due to heavy rains in the mountains. Because the skies were clear over town, many did not evacuate. The warning message conflicted with their own evaluation of the weather. Other residents were told incorrectly that a dam break precipitated the flood. These citizens believed the warning at once. The message did not conflict with their own reading of the signs.[12]

When you give a patient an "emergency warning" about treatment need, your message should match the patient's reading of dental health signs. Make treatment need observable to the patient. Provide multiple signs of the dental condition if possible. Take the patient on a tour of her mouth and say, "See here? . . . and see here?. . . You can see for yourself that . . . ." Explain the relevance of any symptoms the patient may have experienced by saying, "You may have noticed (bleeding gums, sensitivity, eating difficulty, etc.) as symptoms of this condition." X-rays, models, and multimedia computer technology are not just tools for explanation, but tools for persuasion of the need for treatment.

Demonstrate the severity of the problem

After you have shown the symptoms of the dental condition, discuss the long-term effects of the dental problem and describe the impact of the problem on important aspects of the patient's life. For example, "If we remove this tooth instead of fixing it, the teeth around it will shift out of position. This will affect not only the look of your smile, but also your ability to eat and speak effectively."

Describe how the dental health the patient takes for granted is at risk

For example, "You have been used to eating whatever you like, but without treatment you may encounter difficulty eating some of your favorite foods," or "You have had a great track record of keeping every one of your teeth to this point in life. If we don't take care of this gum condition, you face the potential loss of these two teeth right here."

Explain why it's urgent

Patients are more likely to act if they believe that their symptoms should be dealt with promptly. You may need to emphasize to the patient that the problem is particularly acute, requiring treatment immediately. Or, you may need to communicate that the dental situation is deteriorating and the time for action is limited.

Identity: The Secret of Case Acceptance Is a Patient Who Says "I Think I Can"

Patients who take action on treatment believe four things:

1. I understand the seriousness of my dental condition.
2. I know exactly what specific treatment steps will solve the problem.
3. I know the treatment will be effective.
4. I know I am capable of taking action.

Most dental communicators do an admirable job of explaining dental problems, outlining specific steps in treatment plans, and emphasizing the effectiveness of recommended treatments. But the communication technique usually left out—and the one often most essential to case acceptance—is telling patients they are capable of accepting treatment. In fact, research demonstrates that a belief in one's own effectiveness is the most powerful predictor of a healthy lifestyle.[13] How can you promote a patient's sense of personal power?

Tell her she is the type of person who would take action

Sometimes a patient hesitates to accept treatment because she does not consider herself to be the kind of person who invests time and money in dental treatment.[14] Find a characteristic that the patient is willing to attribute to herself and show how that characteristic is related to treatment acceptance. This approach can be summed up as, "Although you may not realize it, you have the ability to achieve good dental health."

For example, a patient who is otherwise healthy but puts off periodontal therapy might react positively to, "A lifestyle as healthy as yours is only possible for someone capable of great personal commitment. That's why I believe you are the kind of person who will go forward with this."

Voice confidence in the patient's abilities

For example, you might say, "I know you will make a wise decision about the treatment," or "Now that your treatment is completed, you are in the driver's seat. I will be riding along with you to give occasional directions about home care."

If the patient believes his dental situation is hopeless, do not try to convince him it's "not all that bad." Instead, acknowledge the difficulty of the situation, then describe specific treatment options still available for his condition. You might mention other patients who faced the same dental problem and reached eventual good health. For example, "I know this is not what you hoped to hear. It is indeed a challenging situation for any patient. Let's discuss the treatment options still possible for you. I had a patient last year who found himself in a similar situation. Extensive though the treatment was, he stayed with it and we were able to save his teeth."

Share control of the treatment process

Participation leads to persuasion. Most people find a plan of action more favorable if they helped develop it, carrying an attitude of "It must be good because I thought of it." As the authors of *Getting to Yes* state, "If people are not involved in the process, they are hardly likely to approve the product. It is that simple. Agreement becomes much easier if both parties feel ownership of the ideas. Participation in the process is perhaps the single most important factor in determining whether a proposal is accepted."[15]

When a patient has an important choice to make about treatment options, consider what information you could provide to assist in the decision. A straightforward description of the two procedures is not enough. A comparison of the advantages and disadvantages of the two treatment alternatives is equally important. Here is a sample outline of an information sheet for a patient who needs to make a decision between amalgam and composite fillings.

Amalgam Fillings	Composite Resin Fillings
Advantages • Affordable, approximately one-half the cost of composites • Durable	Advantages • Natural appearance, virtually invisible
Disadvantages • Cosmetic considerations	Disadvantages • May be less durable, especially on chewing surfaces • Cost considerations

Four Deadly Sins of Case Presentations

If patients are not allowed to "save face" when confronted with a dental problem, they often deny the entire situation.[16] For example, if a mother catches her child with a hand in the cookie jar and accuses the youngster of stealing cookies, the child may actually deny it—even though his hand is still in the jar. People deny reality when under strong external threat. The following four "deadly sins" place excessive pressure on patients, thus leading to possible denial of both the dental problem and the proposed treatment.[14]

1. *Blame.* Blaming patients for causing dental conditions or for failing to deal with dental problems. Example: "I can't believe you let your mouth get in this condition."

2. *Moral superiority.* Taking the approach that if patients don't do what you say, they lack an important moral value. (Translation: They are slime.) Example: "Any responsible parent would make sure their child receives the treatment I recommend."

3. *Sales pressure.* Pushing patients into treatment decisions before they are ready. Example: "Surely you agree that this is the best thing to do. I'm going to tell Susan to schedule you an appointment right now."

4. *Threats.* Using threats of dire dental consequences for the sole purpose of limiting patients' freedom of choice in treatment. Example: "If you don't agree to this treatment now, then you will lose that tooth. You really have no choice at this point."

Here are two ways to lessen the intensity of a patient confrontation on dental habits.[16] First, begin by talking in general to give the patient a chance to make it personal. Example: "A lot of patients tell me they have trouble remembering to floss." Second, build in loopholes for the patient by using such words as "sometimes," "maybe," "once in a while." For example, rather than saying, "You grind your teeth, don't you?" you might say, "It looks like you grind your teeth sometimes."

Value: How to Help Patients Say "I Don't Just Need It, I Want It"

In deciding whether they want to proceed with treatment, patients make a personal assessment of the advantages and disadvantages of the treatment plan. In their own ways, they weigh the pluses and minuses of doing what you suggest, doing something else, or doing nothing. If your proposed treatment has the most pluses and the fewest minuses of the three choices of action, patients are more likely to accept your recommendations. So, this step in persuasion is straightforward: Maximize the advantages and minimize the disadvantages of the proposed treatment compared with the treatment alternatives or no treatment at all.

Emphasize the benefits

Remember that a benefit is not what the treatment is, but what the treatment does. The treatment is a description of the dental service; the benefit is what the service will mean to the patient's quality of life.

People buy benefits, not products or services. For example, people don't buy soap, they buy cleanliness. They don't buy aspirin, they buy freedom from pain. They don't buy cars, they buy mobility. They don't buy life insurance, they buy security and peace of mind.

Similarly, parents don't buy orthodontic appliances for their teens, they buy self-confidence and future dental health for their children. Older adults don't buy dentures, they buy comfort and function when they eat, speak, and smile. Business executives don't buy laminate veneers, they buy an attractive appearance for important client meetings. To truly be persuasive, you must spell out the benefits of treatment and help patients imagine themselves receiving the treatment benefits.

One last benefit of stressing benefits: Patients pay more attention to positive messages than to negative ones. Positive statements are more memorable and more likely to result in behavior change. That's why public health campaigns have turned from such negative approaches as "This is your brain (egg). This is your brain on drugs (fried egg). Any questions?" and employ more upbeat messages as "Just Say No," and "Be Smart—Don't Start."[17]

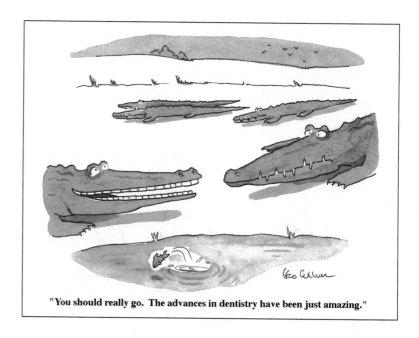

"You should really go. The advances in dentistry have been just amazing."

Deal with the disadvantages

Patients hesitate to accept treatment because of the time, inconvenience, or discomfort involved. (They also hesitate about the cost, which will be discussed in the next chapter.) You have four possible approaches for dealing with the disadvantages of treatment.[14]

The first is explaining how the disadvantages can be minimized. For example, "You're concerned about the visits disrupting your work schedule? That's certainly understandable. Would it help if we scheduled your appointments in the early morning hours?" Or, "You're worried that it might be uncomfortable? Here's how we can make the procedure as comfortable as possible."

A second approach is to compare the disadvantages of treatment with the advantages of treatment. (Of course, the disadvantages will be smaller than the advantages in your comparison.) For example, "Mrs. Jones, I'm not going to tell you that this treatment won't take some time. It will. But when it's completed, you will have a smile to be proud of."

A third approach is to compare the disadvantages of treatment with the disadvantages of no treatment. If possible, show patients that they currently suffer from disadvantages far greater than those posed by the treatment. For example, "Mr. Smith, I recognize that this treatment will put a squeeze on your already busy work schedule. But without the treatment, you may find yourself in an emergency situation that will be far more inconvenient for you."

A fourth approach is to show how the disadvantages of no treatment will increase over time. For example, "If we take care of this now, the treatment can be both affordable and comfortable. If we wait, you will face a greater expense and potential discomfort down the road."

An Outline for Case Presentations

Dental condition

Recommended treatment

Treatment benefits

Treatment risks

Alternate treatments

Results of no treatment

Patient questions

Request for action

Summary

Case Presentation Tips

- Be on time or explain why you aren't.

- Open with one remark geared to the patient as a person, not a dental problem.

- Organize your message around teeth, not around treatments. For example, don't say, "We will do X treatment on this tooth, this tooth, and this tooth. We will do Y treatment here and here." The patient gets confused when you jump around from tooth to tooth in your discussion. Instead say, "Let's talk about this tooth right here. It needs X and Y treatment. Now let's talk about this tooth over here. It will require X and Z treatment."

- Don't refer to teeth by numbers. This reference is lost on patients. Call teeth by name and location such as "the very back molar on your right side."

- Spend less time on treatment specifics and more time on treatment benefits.

- Use more patient examples. Match your examples with the age and gender of the patient.

- Don't use dental charts or X-rays as your primary visual aids. They don't look like real teeth in a person's mouth. Use the patient's mouth or a model as your primary visual, then refer to the X-rays or chart as necessary. For example, "See this tooth on the model? Here it is on your X-ray."

- Humor is fine, but no jokes downgrading yourself, your staff, or the patient. Avoid humor that excludes the patient, such as referring to a funny staff-meeting incident. And, of course, politically incorrect jokes are out.

- Ask for patient questions. Even if you're running late.

- Put it in writing. A written treatment plan will increase your credibility and help patients remember your message after they get home. It also will keep the dental assistant from having to repeat everything you said after you leave the room.

Action: What to Say to the One in Two Patients Who Doesn't Comply

Half of dental patients follow home-care and post-treatment instructions, half don't. To be more specific, about one-third of patients are highly compliant with suggested oral hygiene procedures, one-third comply moderately well, and the remaining third fail to comply.[18] This compliance rate is similar to patient adherence with other medical advice.

When patients don't follow your instructions, your first reaction is that they didn't understand what they were supposed to do. Usually that's not it. More than 70 percent of patient noncompliance is intentional.[19] Following doctor's orders is not simply a matter of understanding the directions. It's also a matter of patient judgment about the worth and difficulty of the treatment instructions.

Here are four reasons patients don't follow treatment instructions, followed by communication techniques to overcome each obstacle to compliance.

Patient Excuse #1: I don't know what to do

Solution: Be specific. A hygienist gave her orthodontic patient a handful of rubber bands and told him to "put a new set on every day." Three days later the patient called and said he couldn't get on any more bands. He'd layered the bands on top of each other, not knowing he was supposed to take the previous ones off. The single most important factor in getting appropriate action is the specificity with which the action is described. For example, you don't ask patients to "take better care of their teeth," you ask them to "brush after breakfast and before bed."

The 1989 San Francisco earthquake offers a compelling example of the importance of specific directions. After the earthquake struck, officials walked the streets of affected areas in downtown San Francisco telling people not just to "make sure you have water" but instead to "fill your bathtub with water." More specific instructions led to more action by Bay area citizens.[20] Another good example of message specificity is the "five a day" campaign to encourage consumers to eat more fruits and vegetables.

Patient Excuse #2: It's too hard

Solution: Make it easy. You give patients reader-friendly lists of post-treatment instructions to place on the refrigerator. (You even supply the magnet.) You furnish toothbrushes, toothpaste, and floss. You hand out miniature hourglasses so patients can time how long they brush. These are all excellent examples of making home care easy.

Another technique is called "foot in the door." In this approach, you ask the patient to take a small initial step, then later add steps requiring more effort or difficulty. What's the reasoning behind this technique? People want to be consistent. If they first perform a relatively trivial action, they are more likely to perform a similar act later that requires greater sacrifice.[21] For example, if you ask a parent to cut down the frequency of sugary snacks for her children, she may judge the action as too difficult. As an initial step, you might ask her to select one low-sugar snack the next time she visits the grocery store. Or, you might ask her to sit down with her children and make a list of low-sugar foods they really enjoy. Note: Because the impact of this type of message dissipates quickly, choose an action that must be performed promptly.

Patient Excuse #3: It doesn't fit into my routine

Solution: Help the patient fit the treatment into daily life. It's easier to ignore instructions than to change lifestyle. Therefore, the harder the directions are to follow on a daily basis, the less likely the patient is to comply.[22] One of the best ways to help patients see exactly when and how home care would fit into their routine is to tie it to something they already do. Examples: "What's your child's evening routine? Great! Then the brushing could fit in between the bath and the book." "You usually watch *Oprah* after breakfast? Maybe you could decide to turn on the TV only after you brush. Then you could floss during the commercials."

Patient Excuse #4: I forgot

Solution: Give them something to jog their memories. A sticker to place above the sink and other reminders really do work.

A Hygienist's Guide to Patient Compliance

Dental compliance research offers the following tips to enhance patient education sessions.[18,23]

- Information alone will not change behavior. Patients will not brush and floss simply on the basis of a comprehensive explanation of the causes of gum disease. Involve patients in both the discussion and practice of good home care.

- Listening is essential. In fact, the amount of time patients speak during plaque-control discussions could be more important than the amount of time you speak.

- The more specific the message, the better the results. Tell patients exactly what they should do when they get home.

- Asking patients to demonstrate their skills is a successful technique. After you have observed a patient's skills, you can target instruction to the individual patient.

- Some patients see education as criticism. Overcome this perception with the message that you hope to improve their efficiency, thus maximizing the benefits they receive from time spent on home care.

- Positive feedback works to increase compliance. Compliment every patient, even if you have to reach for it. A hygienist once said, "You are doing a great job brushing your front four teeth. Now if we could see that same dedication on some other areas of your mouth . . ."

- Positive consequences work to increase compliance as well. Encourage parents to show approval to their children for good brushing and flossing. (Stars on a chart is a time-honored technique because it's successful.) Suggest to adults that they reward themselves with an activity they enjoy, such as renting a movie or visiting a friend.

- Negative messages aren't successful at changing behavior. You may need to discourage some parents from nagging or punishing children for thumb-sucking or other oral habits. To avoid sounding judgmental yourself about a patient's dental habits, you may need to remain admirably restrained in your comments—at least until you reach the staff room and close the door.

- Monitoring behavior is successful for some patients. For example, you might ask patients to check off their home-care actions on a chart and bring the chart with them on the next visit.

- Repeat an important message three times, perhaps in different ways, to make it memorable and to get action.

Questions & Answers

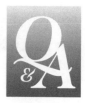

Filling Baby Teeth

"Why do you want to fill baby teeth? They will fall out anyway."

Comment   This parent holds an inaccurate but plausible idea about dental treatment for her child. First acknowledge the parent's views. Then demonstrate the strength of your views by using information familiar to the parent.

Great answer   "I can see why you would wonder about that. It's confusing when some of the teeth we call baby teeth may stay in a child's mouth until he's 12. While it is true that baby teeth do eventually come out, it is also true that they are important to your child in the meantime. Tony needs his baby teeth to speak clearly, eat comfortably, and smile with confidence. Also, his baby teeth are holding space for his permanent teeth. If one is lost, the others shift into the empty space. This often means a crooked smile in a child's future. An investment in treatment now will save Tony from dental problems down the road, including possible infection and discomfort."

Comparing Cavities in Siblings

"How come Tommy gets so many more cavities than Mary when they eat the same things? Tommy must have soft teeth like his dad."

Great answer   "It just doesn't seem fair, does it, when Tommy tries so hard? It seems logical that if they eat the same things and don't get the same number of cavities, then their teeth must be different. But let's take a closer look. There are three reasons Tommy might get more cavities. First, unique physical makeup. Siblings may look and sound alike, but still have a different capacity for dental health. As unfair as it seems, some children do everything right and still get cavities. Second, eating habits. It's not just what a child eats, but how often he eats it. (Explore Tommy's snacking habits with the parent. Mary may eat her candy bar all at once; Tommy may nibble on his during an hour of Nintendo.) Third, brushing and flossing habits. (Tommy's brushing style may be enthusiastic but inefficient.) Let's talk about treatment and home-care possibilities that will help Tommy."

Post-treatment Discomfort _____

"My teeth didn't hurt before I had scaling and root planing. Why do they hurt now?"

Great answer "Of course you're concerned. Your comfort is important. You would think that if you have a problem taken care of, your body should feel better immediately. But with many health conditions, the body hurts more when it's healing than when it's hurt. You've been feeling sensitivity to hot and cold, is that right? You should be feeling more comfortable within 36 hours, but people vary in their response to treatment. Some people have little to no discomfort; others feel discomfort for up to a week. What's important is the trend of the discomfort. Is it getting progressively less? If it stays the same, or gets worse, please let me know. Here are some suggestions to make you more comfortable in the meantime."

Extraction as Treatment Option _____

"My wife says I should just have all my teeth pulled. Her parents did."

Possible answer "If your wife thinks that's such a great idea, perhaps she should have it done first." Or, "What do your wife's parents look like?"

Comment Don't insult the person this patient no doubt refers to as his "better half." Instead, give him an arsenal of arguments for convincing his wife that another treatment option is best. If possible, invite her in for future treatment discussions. She's probably the primary decision-maker for health care in the family.

Great answer "That's one treatment option to consider. What do you think of it? You're not sure? Well, let's talk about exactly what that treatment would mean for you. Then we can talk about your goals for your smile and your other treatment choices, comparing the advantages and disadvantages. There are many treatments available for you that weren't around for your wife's parents."

No Examination by Dentist _____

"Why do I have to have an exam by the doctor? I trust your judgment." (To hygienist after teeth cleaning)

Great answer "I am honored that you trust my judgment. I appreciate your confidence in me. But the dentist is knowledgeable in many areas that a hygienist is not. That's why it's in your best interests to have the dentist examine your teeth as well. A thorough clinical examination will diagnose decay, periodontal disease, and other potentially serious conditions that may require prompt treatment."

Just Treatment, No Examination _____

"I just want to get this tooth filled."

Great answer "Certainly the doctor will fill your tooth and relieve your immediate concerns. But he also will evaluate your overall dental health to diagnose periodontal disease, oral cancer, and other potentially serious conditions that can affect your overall health. I know the lost filling has been inconvenient for you. A clinical examination will help avoid future dental problems like this one."

Postponing Treatment _____

"What will happen if I do nothing?" (Or, "Can I put this treatment off until next year?")

Great answer "That's a reasonable question because some health conditions—like a flu virus, for example—can go away without treatment. But dental conditions aren't like that. Living with the condition doesn't make it go away. It makes it worse. I advise prompt treatment. If we plan what is necessary now, we can restore you to good health. The sooner you have the treatment, the more comfortable and affordable it will be. Most important, if you do nothing, you eventually will lose that tooth. But it is your smile and your decision. Here is a question you may wish to ask yourself: Since I know it's a question of when, not if, I need treatment, will waiting be worth the additional cost and potential for discomfort?"

Need for Fillings _____

"Why do I need these fillings? Nothing hurts."

Possible answer "Because I need the money. Just kidding!"

Comment Feel free to use humor in treatment explanations, but not about dental costs. People think money-related jokes are funny only when the money belongs to someone else. And in the dental office, patients perceive all money as their money.

Great answer "It seems reasonable to wonder if you need to go ahead with treatment when you don't have any symptoms. After all, when you sprain an ankle or have the flu, you know there is a health problem. But tooth decay is like other health conditions—high blood pressure, anemia, or diabetes—that can exist without any symptoms at first. Decay doesn't cause pain until it reaches the pulp or nerve. If we catch decay early, you can avoid pain and possible root canal treatment. In fact, by the time a decayed tooth hurts, it's usually too late to save the tooth with a filling."

Nitrous Oxide _____

"My kid is fine. He doesn't need that gas."

Great answer   "Billy does seem fairly calm right now. But as soon as some unfamiliar noises and sensations occur, he may become anxious. We would like to help Billy to remain calm and have a good visit today. The nitrous oxide helps him relax. He'll be breathing more oxygen than you and I are right now. We'll get the work done faster—probably 20 minutes with the air and 45 or more minutes without the nitrous. Does this information help you with your decision about the air? Do you have any other concerns?"

Need for Recall Visits _____

"Why do I need to come back every six months?"

Great answer   "To maintain your good health through quality care. (You might add: The most precious things in life need regular service, like a fine sports car or a grand piano.) If every six months we examine your mouth and provide an oral cancer screening, we will protect your overall health and dental health. A watchful eye on your health will prevent unpleasant surprises. For example, in this morning's visit, we were able to prevent a tooth from breaking."

Periodontal Retreatment _____

"I've heard that gum treatment doesn't work and has to be done over and over again."

Great answer   "My goal is to avoid 'repeat business.' Although we pride ourselves on providing the highest quality of care possible, the biggest difference between gums that need to be treated again and gums that don't is the person they belong to. It all comes down to home care after the periodontal treatment. I promise to give you all the information and skills you need to keep yourself in top dental health after your treatment."

No Time for Treatment _____

"I don't have time for this right now."

Great answer "It's tough to find time for everything, isn't it? And it's hard to decide what is the best use of your time. Were you wondering how long you could postpone this treatment and what effect it would have on your heath? If you wait, you run the risk of needing more extensive—and more expensive—treatment down the road. The sooner you have the treatment, the more comfortable and affordable it will be. In your decision, you also need to consider the inconvenience of a possible emergency visit. You may find it more time-efficient to schedule a visit than to need an unexpected visit. That's why I advise prompt treatment."

Treatment Discomfort _____

"I know this is going to hurt!"

Comment When team members respond to patient concerns of treatment comfort, the first step is to validate the patient's perspective without echoing negative words from the patient. ("So you're afraid it's going to hurt like hell?") The next step is to find out what particular aspect of treatment worries the patient; it could be something easily solved. The final step is to give personal testimony of the doctor's ability in treatment comfort. Messages to avoid are those offering false promises. If you say it won't hurt and it does, the patient will wonder what else you haven't been completely truthful about.

Great answer "You are concerned the treatment may be uncomfortable? Anything in particular you find bothersome? The initial injection? We can numb the area with a local anesthetic on a cotton ball to make it more comfortable. What else? The light hurts your eyes? Would you like a pair of sunglasses to wear? You know, before I worked in a dental office, I was a very nervous patient. It's helped me to watch the doctor and see how gentle the treatment can be. I have my family treated here, and the doctor has made their visits as comfortable as possible."

"That was awful! If I had known how bad it was going to be, I wouldn't have had the treatment."

Great answer "So you found it more difficult that you expected? Each person has his or her own unique threshold for discomfort, and this is a tough procedure that some patients find uncomfortable. I must compliment you on going ahead with the treatment anyway and sitting through it as well as you did. You made a wise, if difficult, decision that will greatly benefit your health and save your smile. At some point I would like to discuss with you what you can do to prevent the need for this treatment again."

Child Patient Complaints _____

"My Justin said you told him to 'shut up'!" (The parent confronts the dentist with this statement immediately after the visit. You didn't tell Justin to "shut up," you merely wanted to.)

Great answer "How upsetting that must have been to hear! No parent wants their child to be talked to that way! I can assure you I didn't—and would never—say that to a child in this practice. But it's a difficult situation for you when your child says one thing and the other person says something else. What would help you feel more comfortable with all this? My dental assistant was in the room the entire visit. Would you like to speak with her about what happened? The important thing here to me is that Justin was uncomfortable with the dental visit. Could I describe the visit for you, and you could let me know what we might be able to do next time to help Justin feel more relaxed with us?"

Denture Adjustment _____

"Another denture adjustment? I don't understand why it takes so many visits to get it right."

Great answer "I know it's taken more visits than you expected. It has been a long process, and I must thank you for working with us on this. Would it help to have a quick description of what we've accomplished and what's left to complete? I'd be happy to do that. In your particular case, we needed the additional time to reach a high level of comfort for you with your dentures. Each person's body is unique, so each patient requires his or her own special level of care. Is there anything the front desk can do to make the visits at a time more convenient for you?"

Fluoride Treatments _____

"My Sarah hates fluoride treatments. Are they really necessary?"

Comment Your first goal is to show concern for Sarah's discomfort. Your second goal is to find the source of dislike of the treatment; you may be able to adjust the treatment to match the child's preferences. For example, if Sarah hates the taste, you could try a different flavor. If she thinks it takes too long, you could provide a timer for Sarah to watch during the treatment. Your final goal is to stress the benefits of the fluoride treatment for Sarah in particular.

Great answer "So Sarah really dislikes it? It's hard, isn't it, when a child needs a treatment but doesn't like it? Something in particular she doesn't like? (Find the source of dislike; present your ideas on adjusting the treatment.) Do you have any ideas on making the treatment easier? What if she held her stuffed bear or we offered her a special reward? Sarah in particular does benefit from fluoride treatments at each visit to protect her from decay."

Crying Child

"Will the dentist stop treatment if my child cries?"

Great answer "How we handle treatment with your child is entirely your decision. Let's talk about what we have found works best in our experience with children over the years. We will begin by making your child as comfortable as possible. We then make the treatment as gentle as it can be. It has been our experience that, even if a child cries, it's better to proceed with the treatment so the child has a sense of pride at the end of the visit. We want to reward him for bravery. If we stop, the child will not have the sense of accomplishment, will still have the treatment to face at a later date, and will be more likely—rather than less likely—to be upset at a later visit."

Great answer "Yes, we will, but because we keep such a close eye on your child, it seldom gets to that point. We can tell when your child needs a break. Then after the break, we proceed with the treatment. It has been our experience that, even if a child cries, it's better to proceed with the treatment so the child has a sense of pride at the end of the visit. We want to reward him for bravery."

*Dental Analogies for Treatment Explanations**

Sometimes a patient objects to treatment because he doesn't have a clear mental image of what the procedure involves. When that's the case, use communication techniques that paint a picture for the patient, such as analogies or comparisons.

The following analogies may be incorporated into your answers along with the other methods discussed in this chapter. For example, you might acknowledge the patient's concern, explain the steps of treatment, use an analogy, then conclude with the specific benefits of treatment in view of the patient's lifestyle. (In other words, analogies do not stand alone as an answer.) You would, of course, choose an analogy complementary to the age, interest, and personality of the patient. One last point: Do not use analogies with young children. Their oh-so-literal minds become even more confused.

---

*Analogies reprinted with permission from *Dental Analogies* by Drs. Rick Waters and Bill Powell (available through The Levin Group, 1-800-443-3303).

Question "I don't see why you have to fill the inside of the tooth (root canal) if there will be a crown over the whole thing."

Analogy "Look at endodontic therapy as if it were the packing in a cardboard box. If you stood on an empty cardboard box, it would collapse. No empty cardboard box can support very much weight. But, if you packed the box full of books, we both could stand on it. Since the nerve in this tooth is dead and the tooth is now hollow, it must be strengthened from within, much like putting the books in the box."

Question "Those old fillings aren't bothering me. Why not wait to fix them with crowns?"

Analogy "Your large fillings are wearing down and the teeth are losing their support. It's a lot like riding on tread-worn tires. They are still holding air and riding okay, but you would still replace them because any extra miles would be unsafe miles. No one knows how close these teeth are to failure. A crown will help protect that from happening."

Question "Will I have to worry about gum disease after my gum surgery is finished?"

Analogy "In some ways periodontal disease is like diabetes, but not quite as serious. Just as a person with diabetes is forever at risk when eating sweets, you have an increased risk of developing periodontal problems again. That is why it is critical that you pay careful attention to your home care and make regular appointments to help keep disease from developing again."

Question "Why can't I have the crowns and bridge without periodontal therapy?"

Analogy "You would never build a fine home on sandy soil without first developing the best of firm foundations. These bridges and crowns will not hold up to 200-pound chewing forces if attached to weak teeth."

Question "Will I ever get used to my new dentures?"

Analogy "The bulk you notice is the denture replacing teeth, bone, and the gums that are missing. Your tongue and cheeks have to get used to that. When you first learned to walk, you had to pay attention to each step. You fell, sometimes many times. But you got back up and soon were running."

Question Why don't my new dentures feel the same? I'm not sure I'm going to be able to get used to them."

Analogy "The reason your dentures feel different is because they are. They allow for all of the bone and gum changes that have taken place since your last ones were prescribed. You will get used to them in time. It's like driving a new car. At first, you fumble for the light and wiper switches and the radio knob. Soon, you are changing gears, turning on the radio, and setting your cruise control simultaneously."

Question "Why do we have to replace that tooth?"
Analogy "Your teeth are lined up like books on a shelf. If one is removed, the others next to it fall into that newly formed space. Something similar begins the day a tooth is removed."

Skill Summary

When the patient finds dental information hard to understand

- Match your message to the patient's background, knowledge, and interests
- Begin with a preview statement to help the patient create a mental outline of your explanation
- Use short sentences and familiar words
- Involve the patient in the discussion
- Briefly summarize your important points
- Provide written information for the patient to take home

When the patient isn't convinced he really needs the treatment

- Take the patient on a tour of his mouth and point out the signs of the dental condition
- Explain how symptoms the patient may have experienced are relevant to the dental condition
- Describe the impact of the dental condition on the patient's quality of life
- Show how dental health the patient takes for granted is at risk

When the patient doesn't consider herself capable of seeking dental treatment

- Find a characteristic that the patient is willing to attribute to herself, such as commitment to her children or dedication to a healthy lifestyle, and tell how that characteristic is relevant to treatment acceptance
- Voice confidence in the patient's abilities to go forward with treatment
- Involve the patient in treatment decisions

When the patient isn't sure the treatment is worth the time or inconvenience

- Emphasize the benefits of treatment
- Explain how the disadvantages of treatment can be minimized
- Compare the disadvantages of treatment with the greater advantages of treatment
- Compare the disadvantages of treatment with the greater disadvantages of no treatment

When the patient doesn't comply with a home-care program

- Give specific instructions in person
- Make the action easier by providing written take-home instructions, oral health aids, reminder stickers, and the like
- Help the patient see how the home-care program would fit into her daily routine

References

1. Epstein LH, Cluss PA. A behavioral medicine perspective on adherence to long-term medical regimens. J Consult Clin Psychol 1982;50:950–971.

2. DiMatteo MR. The physician-patient relationship: Effects on the quality of health care. Clin Obstet Gynecol 1994;37:149–167.

3. Sykes C. The attack on excellence. Chicago Tribune Magazine, August 27, 1995.

4. Boyd JR, Covington TR, Stanaszek WF, Coussons RT. Drug defaulting, Part I, Determinants of compliance. Am J Hosp Pharm 1974;31:362–366.

5. Consumer research study. Massachusetts Dental Society; November 1993.

6. Waitzkin H, Stoeckle JD. Information control and the micropolitics of health-care: Summary of an ongoing research project. Soc Sci Med 1976;10:263–276.

7. Rankin JA, Harris MB. Patients' preferences for dentists' behaviors. JADA 1985;110:323–327.

8. Geboy MJ. Communication and behavior management in dentistry. Baltimore: Williams and Wilkins; 1985:14–17.

9. Rowan KE. Why rules for risk communication are not enough: A problem-solving approach to risk communication. Risk Analysis 1994;14:365–374.

10. Witte K. Putting the fear back into fear appeals: The extended parallel process model. Communication Monographs 1992;59:329–349.

11. Witte K. Generating effective risk messages: How scary should your risk communication be? In Burleson BR (ed): Communication Yearbook 18. Thousand Oaks, CA: Sage; 1995:229–254.

12. Gruntfest E, Downing TE, White G. Big Thompson flood exposes need for better flood reaction system to save lives. Civil Engineering 1978;78:72–73.

13. Gillis AJ. Determinants of a health-promoting lifestyle: An integrative review. J Adv Nurs 1993;18:345–353.

14. Clark R. Persuasive Messages. New York: Harper & Row; 1984:120–171.

15. Fisher R, Ury W. Getting to Yes: Negotiating Agreement Without Giving In. New York: Penguin Books; 1981:27–28.

16. Gazda GM, Childers WC, Walters RP. Interpersonal Communication: A Handbook for Health Professionals. Rockville, MD: Aspen Publications; 1982:142–143.

17. Monahan JL. Thinking positively: Using positive affect when designing health messages. In Miabach E, Parrot RL (eds): Designing Health Messages. Thousand Oaks, CA: Sage; 1995.

18. Wilson, TG. Compliance: A review of the literature with possible applications to periodontics. J Periodontol 1987;58:706–714.

19. Cooper JK, Love DW, Raffoul PR. Intentional prescription nonadherence (noncompliance) by the elderly. J Am Geriatr Soc 1982;30:329–333.

20. Rowan KE. Goals, obstacles, and strategies in risk communication: A problem-solving approach to improving communication about risks. J Applied Communication Res 1991;19:300–329.

21. Bem DJ. Beliefs, Attitudes and Human Affairs. Belmont, CA: Brooks/Cole; 1970:54–69.

22. Hunt LM, Jordan B, Irwin S, Browner CH. Compliance and the patient's perspective: Controlling symptoms in everyday life. Cult Med Psychiatry 1989;13:315–334.

23. Weinstein P, Getz T, Milgrom P. Oral self-care: A promising alternative behavior model. JADA 1983;107:67–70.

"It Costs How Much?"

Explaining Fees and Dental Benefits

"Money is better than poverty, if only for financial reasons."

—Woody Allen

"If you think you have someone eating out of your hand, it's a good idea to count your fingers."

—Martin Buxbaum

"Why does it cost so much?" "How do you set your fees?" "Why did the insurance company say you're too expensive?" "Why do I have a bill if I have insurance?" "Why haven't you joined the discount dental plan offered by my union?" This chapter offers practical advice on responding effectively to patient questions about dental costs.

Two issues make fee discussions difficult: cost fairness from the patient's perspective and treatment value in view of dental fees. In the first category of tough questions about dental costs, patients want to know if your fees are fair. Have you been honest and ethical in setting fee levels? Are your financial policies even-handed? Could a patient buy exactly the same service from another dentist for a lot less? In the second category of questions, patients want to know if the treatment is worth the cost. Will they get what they pay for? Does the treatment represent a wise investment? Will relevant needs or wants be met in exchange for their expenditure of funds? Specific communication techniques will help you overcome these obstacles to successful fee discussions.

Key Issues in Fee Discussions

Patient issue	Patient examples
Cost fairness	Is this office honest in setting fees? Could I buy the same service from another dentist for less?
Treatment value	Is the treatment worth the price? Will I get something I need or want for my money?

Facts on Fees: Patients Don't Look at Money the Way You Do

Recent consumer research offers insights on how money affects patient actions in the dental office. When choosing your messages on dental care costs, consider the following points.

Although some patients select a dentist on price alone, an equal number don't

In a national Gallup survey commissioned by the American Dental Association, consumers were asked: "If two dentists were in similar locations, and all you knew about them was the fees they charged, would you go to the dentist who charged less?" Forty-seven percent said they would, 31 percent said they would not, and 22 percent said they needed more information than just fees to select a dentist.[1] So in terms of attracting patients to your practice, one-half of your potential market thinks fee levels are very important, and one-half considers other aspects of your practice—such as perceived quality of treatment and dentist rapport—as more central to their decision.

Patients are less afraid of the dentist than of the dental bill

Cost is the top reason people say they put off dental appointments. It's more relevant than pain or fear in avoiding dental visits.

Percentage of consumers*	Reason for avoiding the dentist
50	Can't afford it
27	Afraid
18	Pain
5	Dislike dentists

*This table and the first table on p. 111 are copyright 1991 by the American Dental Association.[1] Reprinted by permission.

Most patients will not switch dentists over price

Dentists on the average have achieved an admirable level of patient loyalty. Most people (90 percent) say that moving out of the area would be the main reason that they would change dentists. Other factors that would make a consumer change dentists are:

Percentage of consumers	Reason for switching dentists
76	Quality of care
62	Rapport with the dentist
47	Cost of dental services

So, although some patients may leave your office in search of lower prices, the majority believe quality relationships and quality treatment are far more important.

Many patients think your fees are reasonable

Consumers respond somewhat favorably on the perceived fairness of dental fees. About 40 percent of consumers rate the fees at dental offices as excellent or good; 40 percent rate them as fair; 20 percent rate them as poor.[1]

The best buys in dentistry are teeth cleaning and pain relief

Although most consumers consider fees reasonable for hygiene services and painful tooth repair, fees for restorative care are perceived as higher than they should be. According to 1993 research from the Massachusetts Dental Society, the following percentages of patients surveyed believed they got their money's worth on the services listed[2]:

Percentage of consumers believing fee was fair	Service
89	Teeth cleaning
82	Treatment of painful teeth
49	Preventive care and fillings
21	Other restorative care

Dental insurance is important to patient decisions

The good news is that patients with dental benefits go to the dentist more often because of their coverage. The bad news is that almost two-thirds of consumers say they would switch dentists if necessary to retain insurance coverage. One-half say they make treatment decisions based on dental benefits.[2]

Trust: It's Not Just the Size of the Fee But the Fairness of It

Why do patients call around for prices? Not only to get a bargain, but to gain information on whether a dental fee is equitable. Why do patients get upset when an insurance company tells them that your fees are not "usual, reasonable, and customary"? Because it sounds as if your fees aren't fair.

People want to know if they are paying a reasonable price for what they are buying, whether it is a car, computer, college education, or porcelain crown. But patients don't have the technical know-how to judge a dental fee in terms of the expertise or materials required for the treatment. Their chief way to measure the equity of dental costs is to measure your character. To trust your fee, they must first trust you.

Chapter 3 provides communication methods for building patient trust in you and your practice in general. Here are skills for building patient trust in the fairness of your fees in particular.

Put it in writing

One way patients decide if a fee or a financial policy is fair is whether it applies to everyone. If you put your financial policies in writing, you strengthen the image that you treat all patients the same way (and thus equitably) in money matters. List financial policies in your practice brochure, provide a financial policy statement as part of your case presentation materials, and describe your financial policy for new patients in welcome letters.

As you already know, giving patients a written financial policy doesn't mean they read it. Increase the importance of your written statements with such spoken messages as, "Here's a copy of the financial policy for our practice. Let me circle the part that's relevant to your treatment. You may want to keep it for your files."

Communicate equity

Suppose a new patient calls to make an appointment. Rather than saying, "You'll need to pay for the visit when you come in," it's better to say, "Our office policy is to ask new patients to cover the cost of dental services at the time they are provided." Such statements as "our office policy is" and "we expect all our patients" communicate that the patient is not being singled out for an unusual (and thus unfair) approach to fees.

Does this mean you can never make exceptions? Certainly not. But when you do make an exception, make sure the patient knows the policy as well as the exception. You might say, "Our financial policy is (X) but I'm giving you an exception this once due to your special circumstances. We would never want to see anyone's health affected because of financial reasons."

Avoid surprises

Another way to prove financial fairness is inform as you perform. When the patient knows about fees and financial policies in advance—rather than finding out too late to consider them in treatment decisions—the process always seems more fair.

Separate the treatment and payment discussions

In an ideal case presentation, the dentist provides a complete explanation of recommended treatment—and leaves the room. The business manager for the practice then explains the fees for

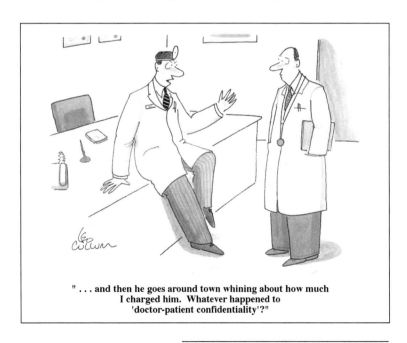

" . . . and then he goes around town whining about how much
I charged him. Whatever happened to
'doctor-patient confidentiality'?"

treatment, reviews financial policies, and offers a choice of payment options. If you use this two-person approach, a patient is more likely to say, "I need the treatment," instead of "The doctor needs the business."

Explain how you arrived at the treatment fee

When a patient receives a written treatment plan, it should include a separate fee for each service or category of service instead of just a total amount for all the services. The business manager can then walk the patient through each dental service and its corresponding fee, answering patient questions in the process.

Be clear, not confusing

People distrust what they don't understand. When patients are faced with such complex concepts as deductibles, copayments, pre-authorizations, and URCs, they may find insurance discussions as confusing as the most clinical of treatment explanations. Remember to:

- Start with a preview statement to give the patient a mental outline of your message
- Put your most important points first and last to make them more memorable
- Use short sentences
- Select familiar words whenever possible
- Define unfamiliar terms
- Highlight key messages through your delivery style
- End with a summary statement

Keep an open door on communication

Nothing damages patient trust in fee fairness more quickly than a perception of limiting access to price information. Although you needn't encourage patients to compare prices with other offices, don't criticize them for gathering fee information on their own. You might say, "It sounds like you've been doing some research into this, and I would never discourage you from doing so. We want you to be comfortable with our fees. I would suggest, though, that you find out exactly what is—and isn't—included in the other fees so that you can make a wise comparison." Or you could say, "Whatever your decision, please don't make it solely on the basis of price. Comfort, convenience, and quality are important as well."

Sample Financial Policy Statements

You may wish to adapt one or more of the following statements for the financial policy of your practice.

General Fee Information

- The best way to save on dental costs is prevention plus quality dentistry as soon as dental problems arise.
- We expect payment from our new patients at the time of the visit, regardless of dental benefits coverage. We accept cash, checks, and credit cards.

Payment Arrangements

- Payment in full at the start of treatment with cash or a check earns a complimentary discount of five percent.
- This practice accepts the following credit cards:
- Patients may prefer to make arrangements with a bank or credit union for the amount of the treatment, making monthly payments to the lending institution.
- For our patients without dental insurance, we require 50 percent of the total fee at the start of treatment. The balance will be due on a 60-day payment schedule.
- Finance charges are added to accounts every 30 days at 1.5 percent of the unpaid balance.

Dental Benefits

- We promise to base your treatment on your dental health needs, not on your insurance policy.
- Although you have insurance coverage, some procedures may not be covered. A deductible or a copayment may be required. Our business manager will be happy to review your dental benefits coverage with you.
- For our patients with insurance, we will be pleased to assist in filing a pre-authorization with the dental insurance company. Payment of the deductible and 50 percent of the copayment is required at the start of treatment. Any balance will be due on completion of the treatment.
- Your level of insurance coverage is determined by the policy your employer selects. If you think your coverage is insufficient, you may wish to address this with your employer.

Value: It's Not the Fee But the Worth of the Treatment

While some patients judge a fee based on whether it seems fair, others judge a fee based on whether they will receive a service equal in value to the money spent. Therefore, when a patient says, "The treatment is too expensive," what the patient may mean is, "The price seems too high for the value received." The issue is not cost, but cost compared with the fulfillment of a need or want. Your communication goal is not to lower the price, but to raise the value of the treatment from the patient's perspective.

Although some dentists advertise low prices as a way to market their practices, price is never a benefit. It's always an objection. People don't buy something because of a low price. People buy something because they want it and the price seems to offer value for their money. Here are ways to enhance the perceived worth of treatment in comparison with the fee.

Document the severity of the dental condition

If patients are not convinced that they need the treatment, they will not be convinced that the treatment is a good investment. Provide evidence of the seriousness of the patient's dental problem with such visuals as X-rays, models, and computer-generated images. Compare the patient's current dental condition with the advantages of good dental health.

Compare the costs with the benefits of treatment

To be persuasive in fee discussions, you must be ready to tell patients what they will get for their money. Describe what the dental treatment will mean to the patient's quality of life in terms of function, appearance, and good health.

Describe how the treatment will save money in the future

One of the most persuasive advantages of dentistry is that virtually every service is designed to reduce dental costs in the long run. For example, "Mrs. Knock, I recognize that this treatment represents a sizable investment for you. But taking care of this now will save you from much larger dental expenses in the future."

Explain how the costs can be made more manageable

If you can show patients how payment difficulties can be minimized, you will help them see that they are capable of paying for treatment. For example, "You're concerned that the fee will pose financial stress on your family, is that correct? Thank you for being honest with me. We have three options for financial arrangements with our patients. Why don't I describe them, then we can talk about which one would best meet your needs."

Financial Discussion Tips

What not to say	What to say instead
How would you like to pay?	Will that be cash, check, or credit card?
Will you be taking care of the amount that the insurance company doesn't?	The fee for your dental treatment will be $1,520. Your dental benefits plan will cover $1,050. The remaining $470 is due at your next visit.
What kind of payment plan did you want?	Our office has three choices of financial arrangements. Which one is best suited to your particular situation?

Questions & Answers

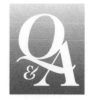

Setting Fees

"Prices vary a lot between dental offices. How do you set your fees?"

Possible answer   "Our fees are variable, based on time plus materials multiplied by the degree of difficulty."

Comment   This answer sounds like one a contractor would give when asked about the price of putting up a new garage. It does not reflect the level of quality health care in your practice.

Another answer submitted in my research was, "First we stammer, then we talk about our overhead, OSHA regulations, stuff like that." This message has such a small potential for success, it's not worth trying. Patients are convinced that dental offices make tons of money. You can't sway them from this notion. Even if they listen to the details of your high overhead, they will not feel particularly sympathetic. Instead, focus on what patients receive for their investment.

Great answer   "Our fees are based upon our ability to provide the highest quality of care available with the best materials and careful adherence to infection control standards. But let's talk about what you receive from your recommended treatment in particular." (Then discuss such treatment benefits as a more attractive smile or the ability to eat more comfortably.)

Great answer   "Your investment is based upon our care, skill, and judgment and the time necessary to provide a high level of service. Here's a copy of your recommended treatment with a fee noted for each service. Let's go over it together." (Then discuss each phase of treatment, comparing the cost with the benefits.)

High Fees

"The cost is so high!"

Possible answer   "I understand how you feel. The money is overwhelming."

Comment   This dental communicator attempts to validate the patient's point of view. But doing so casts a negative light on the fee levels of the dental office. When a patient expresses concern about fees, use the approach recommended in Chapter 3 called "voice the value." (The patient's value is not just receiving a low price, but knowing what he is paying for and getting a good value for his investment.) This approach will allow you to empathize with the patient's perspective while still getting a positive start in your answer.

And as with all patient comments, you need to discover the underlying hesitation of that particular patient. Is the patient unconvinced of the value of treatment? Or, is he convinced of treatment worth but isn't sure how he will pay for it?

Great answer "It is a significant investment. Naturally, you want to be sure you are getting a good value. Are you concerned that the fee is too high for the recommended treatment, or is the amount of the fee difficult for you right now?" (The patient says he has the money but isn't sure the treatment is really worth the price.) "Thank you for being honest with me. You deserve to know precisely what you are paying for. Perhaps the best way I can help you in your decision is to review the benefits of having the treatment and the risks of not having it. By going ahead with the procedure, you will (list of treatment benefits). You will prevent potentially expensive dental problems in the future such as (risks of no treatment). And in terms of appearance, the treatment will put you on your way to a smile anyone would be proud of."

Higher Fees than Another Practice _____

"My husband's dentist doesn't charge that much for a crown. What makes yours so special?"

Great answer "That's an excellent question. Of course you want to make sure you are getting a good value for your investment. I would be pleased to explain what makes your crown so special. First, we have selected the finest materials for your crown. (Continue with other special benefits of the recommended treatment.) You know, most people quite reasonably think that all crowns are alike. But every crown is different, uniquely designed for a specific patient's needs. That's the main reason you see a difference in cost."

Treatment Not Affordable _____

"I can't afford the treatment right now."

Great answer "And it's a sizable investment. It's hard to decide, isn't it, how to best spend our money for the benefit of ourselves and our families? Perhaps I can make your decision clearer by talking about what may happen to your health and your budget if you decide to wait. The longer you wait for treatment, the greater the risk of needing to treat the tooth with a crown instead of a filling. You also face the possibility of an inconvenient emergency situation if the filling breaks, or discomfort if the tooth becomes infected. Would you like to hear about our financial options that make affording dental care easier for many of our families?"

Price Shoppers

"I'm calling around for prices. How much is a filling?"

Possible answer "What kind of filling do you need? You don't know? We provide fee information only after the doctor's clinical examination to determine your need for treatment."

Comment The hidden message in this answer is, "Since we have established that you are clueless about dentistry, why don't you come in and let the real experts take over?" You need a less confrontational way to communicate the message that treatment fees are based on treatment needs, determined only through a clinical examination of a patient's condition.

Great answer "I'll be happy to give you a range. Our fees on file for fillings range from (lowest fee) to (highest fee). That's a big range, isn't it? There are many different types of fillings, since each one is designed to meet the unique dental needs of the patient. Only the doctor can determine the type of filling that is exactly right for you after a careful examination. Please feel free to call other offices for costs, but as you do, I urge you not to make your decision solely on the basis of price. Comfort, quality, and convenience are important as well. May I send you a brochure about our caring approach to patients?"

Exam Fee

"Why do I have to pay for the dentist to examine me? He didn't do anything!"

Comment A friend of mine once called me and said, "I just heard a dentist speak about periodontal problems at my women's club meeting. My dentist has never examined me for gum disease. Should I find a new dentist?" I said, "Call your dentist and talk to him. I'll bet he examines you for gum disease but doesn't describe it as such." She called her dentist, and sure enough, he conducted a careful periodontal examination at each visit, but didn't say anything about the exams because she didn't have periodontal problems.

This dentist's treatment was far better than his talk about treatment. As a result, he came close to losing her (and her husband and three children) as patients. If the professionals at your front desk often hear that "the dentist didn't do anything," then the dentist must step up communication efforts during the clinical examination. Front desk messages should complement information the patient has already heard during the exam itself.

Great answer "You're wondering what value you gain from the doctor's exam? In a clinical examination, the doctor diagnoses not just tooth decay and gum disease, but looks for signs of potentially serious health conditions including bone infections and oral cancer. It's the most important part of preventive dentistry, which means keeping you healthy and your dental costs affordable. Looked at that way, the exam is a great investment."

"My son's exam costs $26? It only took two minutes!"

Great answer "You're right. We are quick. Kids like quick and Jimmy was so cooperative. But the question is: Can we be quick and still be comprehensive? The doctor examined Jimmy for tooth decay and gum disease, as well as for symptoms of other potentially serious health conditions. He observed tooth eruption and growth in view of your child's dental age. You've made an excellent investment in prevention that will save you money in the long run."

Behavior Management Fee _____

"Why do you charge a fee for behavior management for my child?

Great answer "You deserve to know what benefits your child receives for the additional charge. We want to help Brittany be as comfortable and relaxed as possible and to provide the treatment only when she's ready. To meet her special needs, we will need to use extra time and staff, premedication, and special monitoring equipment."

Great answer "The treatment that Brittany so desperately needed required premedication as well as additional staff, time, and expertise. As a comparison, the treatment alternative could have been hospitalization, meaning a difficult experience for Brittany and a serious expense for you. We are glad we were able to complete the treatment here. Brittany was a big help in that."

Senior Discounts _____

"Why can't you offer lower fees to us elderly patients on fixed incomes?"

Comment If your answer is, "We do," then this is not a tough question. The following answer is for those practices that do not offer discounts to all patients-of-record over age 65.

Great answer "We agree that any elderly patient who is financially disadvantaged should not be denied dental care because of the cost. That's why we participate in our state dental society access program. This program provides reduced-fee dentistry to people over age 65 who qualify. We believe this is the best way we can serve those in our community who are most in need. Would you like the telephone number of the dental society to determine your eligibility for the program?"

Fees Higher Than in the 1960s _____

"Thirty years ago a filling cost one-third that much."

Great answer "There's no question that everything costs more these days. The fee increases in dentistry are about the same as increases in other goods and services, from cars and mortgages to groceries and dry cleaning. They have simply kept pace with inflation. (Optional: This is in contrast with medical care, which has increased far more over the years than patients' incomes.) Because we have had phenomenal advancements in our materials and techniques, we offer more to patients dollar-for-dollar than ever before. For example, thirty years ago, you would not have had the choice of a filling that is virtually invisible."

Bill the Father _____

"Please bill the child's father for the treatment."
(divorced mother)

Great answer "Gee, I wish we could. We have found ourselves in this triangle situation before, and have found the best way to handle it is to ask the parent who brings the child in to cover the costs of the visit."

Great answer "I understand the situation is difficult. But so your child's health isn't affected by financial matters, our office policy is: The parent who brings the child in for the appointment is responsible for payment."

No Checkbook _____

"I forgot my checkbook. And my charge cards."

Great answer "I can understand that happening on occasion. Let me give you a self-addressed, stamped envelope addressed to my attention here at the office. Please place your check in the envelope and drop it in the mail by tomorrow at the latest. I will note in my book that we should expect the check by Thursday."

Dentist's New Lexus

"I saw the doctor's new car. You must be doing really well."

Comment   Another variation on this theme is the patient who sees the new carpeting in reception and says, "Nice carpet! Which corner did my crown pay for?" Although patients rib you about new purchases, many believe that wealth equals success equals ability. In other words, if you are doing well, you must be a good dentist. So patients may tease you about a new car, but if you drove around in a rusty station wagon with a dragging muffler, they would wonder what's wrong. Therefore, your message is that you are doing well, thanks to the dedication and loyalty of your patients.

Great answer   "Thank you, we are, actually. Our patients have been dedicated about going ahead with the care they need and have been kind enough to refer their friends and family to us. We feel lucky to serve such fantastic people in our community."

Limited Dental Benefits

"I have insurance. Why do I have a bill?"

Possible answer   "Our fees are fair. The insurance company only pays a certain percentage and the rest is the patient's liability."

Comment   Sounds defensive, doesn't it? Claiming fee fairness without proof or explanation does little to build patient confidence. (Also, don't use the word "liability" in patient conversations. Its primary connotation is legal problems.)

Possible answer   "You are really lucky to have dental insurance. But it's not designed to cover the whole amount, only to be a helping hand in paying for care."

Comment   There are two problems with this answer. First, few patients hearing it will be convinced to feel "lucky." Second, it puts you on the side of the insurance company instead of the patient. You need an answer that clearly puts you where you belong—on the patient's side as an advocate for quality care.

Great answer   "You have every reason to be concerned when it seems as if you are not getting the type of dental benefits you deserve. We have consistent fees for our services, but the many insurance companies out there vary in their payments. Some pay for dental care in full; some do not. We help you file your insurance claims to get the most benefits possible; you are then responsible for the remainder of the fee. If you're unhappy with your dental insurance, you might want to talk to your employer about why they chose a plan that doesn't cover the full fee for this treatment."

"As long as my insurance pays for it, just do everything."

Great answer "Unfortunately, insurance will only pay a portion of the cost. The latest information we have on your insurance plan shows that approximately $400 will be covered. Let's file a pre-authorization to discover more specifically what will be taken care of by your benefits package and what portion you will be responsible for. We don't want any surprises. In the meantime, it is important that you understand your dental condition and the benefits of the treatment so that you can make a wise decision about your dental health."

Negative Explanation of Benefits _____

"Why did the insurance company say you are too expensive?"

Great answer "It's confusing to hear that information from an insurance company. Of course you want to make sure you are receiving a good value for your investment at our office. What the insurance company meant was that it's their job to cover bargain care. Our job is to give you the best care. That's why you see a difference between the care you receive and the care the insurance company pays for."

If the patient needs more information, you might add: "The dental benefits plan that your employer bought for you decides what it will and will not cover. Naturally, the more services they cover—and the higher the fee schedule—and the higher the insurance company's profit margin—the more the plan costs your employer. Perhaps you might wish to talk to the benefits manager at your firm about how much you would value a comprehensive dental benefits package. In the meantime, we will do everything we can to get you all the benefits possible from your insurance plan."

Sealants Not Covered _____

"Why doesn't the insurance company pay for sealants?"

Great answer "That's an excellent question, since sealants offer such wonderful benefits to your child. Some insurance companies cover sealants as a part of the package that's funded by employers; some do not. I'd be happy to give you a brochure about sealants to pass on to the benefits manager at your company. Perhaps it will help encourage them to include sealants the next time they negotiate a dental benefits package."

Not in Capitation Plan _____

"Why haven't you joined the XYZ capitation dental plan?"

Possible answer   "I cannot deliver the quality of care I do now if I am forced to accept lower fees."

Comment   A dangerous answer for two reasons. First, it ties a particular dental plan to quality of care. As your attorney will tell you, you run the risk of legal difficulties. Second, it gives the impression that you provide quality dentistry only when paid to do so.

Great answer   "That's a reasonable question. Why haven't we joined a plan that sounds like a good deal for our patients? We believe that your treatment should be based on your needs, not your insurance coverage. We also believe that you and your doctor, not an insurance company, should decide your treatment. We've reviewed the different approaches to dental benefits out there and believe that other plans do a better job of respecting and protecting your relationship with your doctor." You might add: "Some of our patients have been offered that plan and have opted out of it. They found that their share of the plan's dental premium would cost them more than two dental visits they typically need in a year."

Not a Preferred Provider _____

"I really like it here, but I'll get a discount if I switch to a dentist on this preferred provider list."

Comment   Again, your answer cannot tie a particular plan to quality of care. Instead, point to convenience, continuity, and the comfort of a familiar setting as good reasons for staying with your practice. In addition, leave the door open for patients if they decide to return to your practice in the future.

Great answer   "Thank you! We're glad you are happy here. We value you as a patient. But how do you decide if switching is best for your family and your budget? Please consider these aspects in your decision. First, what does the fine print say on the insurance agreement? Do you know exactly what is covered and what isn't? Second, how convenient are the doctors on the list? Will they provide the care you have come to expect and value? Third, how will your family react to switching to a different dental practice? Whatever your decision, please don't make it solely on the basis of cost. Think about convenience, comfort, and continuity of care as well. Finally, if you decide to switch and you aren't happy, we would certainly welcome you back."

Missed Appointment Charge _____

"I can't believe I was charged $40 for a missed appointment!"

Comment   What's the primary reason behind charging for missed appointments? It is not to collect the nominal charge, but to prevent cancellations without notice. For example, some restaurants now require charge cards to confirm dinner reservations, informing customers that they will be charged in the event of a no-show without a prior cancellation. The policy has reduced cancellations for some restaurants from 40 to 15 percent, even though no-show customers are seldom charged the cancellation fee.[3]

Since the reason behind charging for missed appointments is to prevent cancellations, your staff should be granted leeway to waive the charge for patients who don't normally cancel. For example, if a loyal patient calls to say that she must miss her appointment because her child is very ill, your receptionist can say, "I'm so sorry to hear Jason is sick. Tell him we hope he feels better soon. May I call you tomorrow to reappoint?"

Patients must be notified of your office policy of charging for missed appointments *before* they actually miss one. For example, describe the policy in your practice brochure or welcome letter to new patients. Practice management consultant Jennifer de St. George recommends this message: "As long as we receive 24 hours advance notice of your need to change an appointment, there will be absolutely no charge. However, if something should occur to prevent you from contacting us, there will be a $50 charge for each half hour not used."[4]

Great answer   "We missed you! It's unfortunate when the unforeseeable occurs. We pride ourselves on keeping our costs affordable for patients. One way we do that is efficient use of equipment and professional staff. When a time is reserved for a patient and he or she is unable to use it, we charge a nominal cancellation fee of $40 when we do not receive 24 hours advance notice. I'm going to waive it in your case this time." (Then send the patient a bill for the missed appointment with "waived" written or stamped on it. If the patient misses another appointment without notice, use the same basic message—but charge the cancellation fee.)

Skill Summary

To build patient trust in the fairness of your fee

- Put the financial policies of your practice in writing and distribute them to patients through new patient letters and practice brochures.

- Communicate fee and financial policy information to patients before they are asked to make decisions about treatment.

- Keep treatment discussions separate from payment discussions.

- Provide written treatment plans that include separate fees for individual services as well as total amounts for all services.

- Do not criticize patients for gathering fee information on their own or comparing fees with other offices.

To raise the perceived value of treatment for patients

- Explain carefully the seriousness of dental conditions and discuss the impact of dental problems on oral health, total health, and quality of life.

- Describe the benefits of dental treatment in terms of function, appearance, and good health.

- Explain how dental treatment can save money in the long run.

- Make dental costs manageable through financial arrangements.

References

1. Dentistry in the 90's: Consumer Attitudes and How They Affect Your Practice. Chicago: American Dental Association, Department of Marketing and Seminar Services; 1991.

2. Consumer research study. Massachusetts Dental Society; 1993.

3. Dining Out. Chicago Tribune; March 3, 1996; Section 1:16.

4. de St. George J. Getting Paid for What You Produce. Las Vegas: American Dental Association Annual Session; October 10, 1995.

"What's the Policy?"

Protecting Patient Relationships in Reception

"A well-informed employee is the best salesperson a company can have."

—E.J. Thomas

Questions in reception fly from all directions on all topics from all kinds of people. Front desk professionals face such issues as:

Trust: "Do you bring your own kids here?"

Safety: "Does this office follow infection guidelines with everyone?"

Understanding: "I have an appointment today but I have no idea what it's for."

Persuasion: "Sometimes I wonder if the treatment's worth all this trouble."

Cost: "I can't believe I'm writing a check for this much money!"

Insurance: "I can never remember the difference between a deductible and a copay."

The communication challenges in reception are so diverse that to do them justice, this chapter would have to recap the whole book. In the interests of saving you time, the chapter will focus on those challenges different from communication elsewhere in the dental office. First, reasons why a patient's experience in reception is essential to the success of your practice. Second, checklists for creating a positive first impression for your office. Third, suggestions for professional dress, since appointment coordinators and business managers typically do not wear dental uniforms. Fourth, tips for communicating by telephone, since it's an essential marketing tool for the practice.

A Positive Experience in Reception Is Essential to Practice Success

Picture this practice image: An office sign with a missing letter. A frowning receptionist who can't find the patient's appointment information. Torn, dated magazines and a coffee stain on the reception room table.

Picture this practice image: An easy-to-find office building with free parking. A smiling receptionist who greets the patient by name. An impeccably clean reception room with a vase of fresh flowers.

The two practices described may each provide quality dental services, yet the initial impression is very different. Patients' perceptions would lead them to believe that the second practice has the better doctor.

Your image as a caring professional is created almost instantly in a patient's mind. Some research suggests that people decide whether or not to continue a relationship in the first *three to five minutes* of contact.[1] Patients may decide whether or not they like a practice before they meet the doctor.

Not only do people form first impressions quickly, but they hold fast to those impressions, often in spite of evidence to the contrary. Additional information about another person is interpreted within—or forced to fit—a first impression.[2] In effect, people make up their minds about others upon early acquaintance, and don't like to be proven wrong. Thus, the tone of an entire dental visit can be determined by the first few minutes in reception.

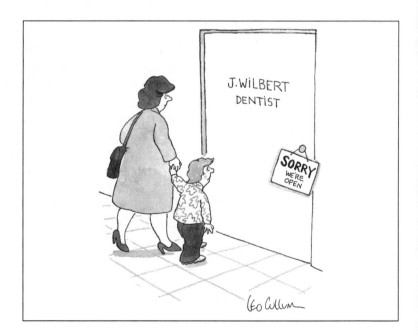

For example, a new patient faces confusion at the front desk about the scheduling of his appointment. An image of inefficiency is set. Conversely, a new patient is greeted graciously by name, told "The doctor is looking forward to meeting you," and escorted promptly to a treatment area. An image of caring efficiency is set.

How can you create a positive first impression for your practice? Let the following two checklists be your guide.

Checklist for Office Entrance and Reception Area

√ The office is clearly marked for both car and pedestrian traffic.

√ The parking area is well-lit, well-maintained, and offers sufficient parking space for patients.

√ The office grounds are attractively landscaped and maintained.

√ The building has a covered entrance.

√ The building lobby is attractive and clean.

√ The dental office entrance is clearly marked.

√ The dental office entrance has a boot mat and ample space for coats, umbrellas, and other patient belongings.

√ The reception area has comfortable seating for patients of all ages.

√ The dental office has a children's play area, stocked with interesting books and toys.

√ The reception area offers a scrapbook of testimonials and thank-you letters from patients.

√ Patient education materials on a variety of dental topics are attractively displayed in the reception area.

√ The reception area offers current reading material for patients of varied interests and ages.

√ The reading material is located neatly in a rack instead of scattered on tables.

√ The reception area has comfortable, attractive, up-to-date furniture.

√ The artwork on reception area walls is attractively framed and appropriately professional.

√ The reception area has ample incandescent (not fluorescent) lighting.

√ The entire reception room area is immaculate.

√ The reception area has healthy plants or fresh flowers.

√ Front office staff have an unobstructed view of the reception room from their work areas.

√ Front office staff have ample counterspace.

√ The office offers a separate space where patients can have private financial discussions.

Checklist for Reception Skills

√ I am familiar with every type of service offered by the practice.

√ I review the medical/dental history form for each patient scheduled for the day.

√ I know the correct pronunciation of each patient's name scheduled for the day.

√ I greet each patient by name, using surnames instead of first names until invited to do otherwise.

√ I provide proper introductions of patients to team members.

√ I inform patients of any necessary waiting time before they ask.

√ I make patients comfortable with the offer of current reading material or refreshments.

√ I check on new information for patient records.

√ When appropriate and natural, I compliment patients.

√ My answers to patient questions are complete but brief.

√ I communicate a message of quality care to each patient.

√ I refrain from eating in front of patients.

√ I establish eye contact with each patient when he or she enters the practice.

√ I sit erect in my chair. (I never slump.)

√ I stand and move with confidence.

√ I seldom lean on or hang over the front desk.

√ I smile a lot (more than I feel like sometimes).

√ I have a firm, confident handshake.

√ I am impeccably groomed.

You Are What You Wear

Should people be judged by how they look? In all fairness, no. Are people judged by how they look? Yes. The following guidelines will assist appointment coordinators, business managers, and other front office professionals in presenting an appearance consistent with a quality dental practice.

Guidelines for Professional Dress

Clean hair styled in a simple manner to stay off the face

Well-fitting glasses (glasses worn on a necklace chain are fine)

Makeup enhancing one's natural appearance

Name tag with first and/or last name

Well-fitting business clothing, such as a tailored dress, or a blazer worn over a blouse and skirt or dress pants

Clothing that is pressed, cleaned, and repaired

Clothing that is more conservative than seductive

Jewelry that stays quiet and in place

Standard-length nails with no polish or polish in standard colors

Well-maintained dress shoes

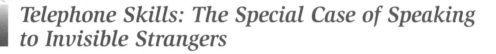

Telephone Skills: The Special Case of Speaking to Invisible Strangers

How to begin

Answer the telephone in two rings or less. (If this is frequently impossible, then the practice needs additional assistance at the front desk.) Identify first the office, then yourself. For example, you might say, "Doctors' Stein and Waters office. This is Rebecca. How may I help you?" Speak with a smile in your voice. (Keep a small mirror on your desk so you can check to see if you are smiling.)

When you don't recognize the caller

If the caller does not identify himself as a current patient or a new patient, ask, "When was your last appointment with us?" By using this approach, the new patient will identify himself as such, and the patient-of-record will not be insulted that you didn't recognize him.

When it's a new patient

When you discover the caller is a new patient, say, "Thank you for calling and welcome to our practice." To obtain information you need from new patients, begin with, "So that we may better prepare for your visit, may I ask you a few questions?" When you have gathered the required information, ask, "Is there anything else we should know to make your visit more comfortable?" Be sure to give each new patient directions to your office, and ask them to bring any relevant information on health status, prescription medication, and insurance coverage.

Rather than asking the new patient, "How did you hear about us?" ask, "Whom may we thank for referring you?" If the new patient was referred by a current patient, say something pleasant such as "Mr. Vernon is an excellent patient," or "I always enjoy seeing Mrs. Schmutzer." If the new patient picked your name at random out of the phone book, say, "That's surprising. This is a mainly a referral practice with satisfied patients telling others about us." Close with, "Do you have any friends or family who would like to join you?"

To arrange appointments

If a patient is calling for an appointment, say, "What may I record as your reason for the appointment?" or "What may I tell the doctor is the reason for the appointment?" It's far more positive than asking, "Why do you want the appointment?" or "What trouble are you having?"

To schedule the appointment, ask, "Do you have a scheduling preference regarding days of the week or mornings versus afternoons?" Attempt to meet the preference with statements such as "Would 3:00 P.M. on Tuesday be convenient?" or "Would 10:00 A.M. on Wednesday suit your needs?"

When you can't hear the patient

Don't say, "What?" or "I can't hear you!" Say instead, "I'm having trouble hearing you. Would you repeat that, please?" Or you might say, "May I double-check that information?"

When you need to place the patient on hold

Ask before you put a patient on hold ("May I put you on hold, please?") and wait for their answer. Check back every two minutes or less. Instead of apologizing, thank the patient for holding. Ask if the patient prefers to continue on hold or to leave a number for a call back.

When the caller is upset

Begin by letting the angry patient blow off steam. Listen attentively to identify the patient's perspective on the problem. Don't interrupt with questions, explanations, or defensive statements. Just say "um-hum" or "please go on" to let them know you're still on the line.

Next, acknowledge the patient's perspective by restating her point of view. For example, "So you expected to feel better by now, but your mouth is still very uncomfortable. Is that right?" Or, "You received a letter from a collection agency, and you are sure it's in error. Is that what happened?" This step will build rapport, clarify problems, and calm anger.

Ask for the patient's help in recording all the information required for an accurate account of the problem. For example, you might say, "I want to make sure I get everything exactly right when I talk to the doctor about this. I'm going to write down your concerns. Would you tell me again what the collection agency said when you called them?"

Because you probably want to give the caller time to calm down further, let him know that you need to check with the doctor (or the insurance company, specialty office, hospital billing department, etc) and call him back. This approach is effective even if you have all the necessary information in front of you. Say, "I very much want to help with this unfortunate situation. I will call you back this afternoon. Is your work or home number best?" Then do call back.

If the caller becomes abusive or your self-control slides toward a desperate urge to scream, try one of these statements: "I really want to help with this, but I'm finding it difficult when you talk to me in this manner." "This isn't going as well as I had hoped. Can I have just a moment to take a deep breath, and then can we start over?" "I'm sorry, but I'm getting too upset to be a very good listener. That's not fair to you. May I call you back in five minutes?"

How to end

Say, "Thank you for calling," and hang up after the patient does. End with "good-bye," not "bye bye."

Questions & Answers

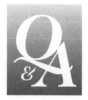

Health History Forms _____

"Why do I have to fill out a health history update?"

Possible answer "It will only take a few moments to complete the form. Something could have changed that we need to know."

Comment Don't start an argument you can't win. The patient thinks the paperwork is a pain. By responding with "it will only take a few moments," you are saying the paperwork is *not* a pain. You can't win this argument. You may find yourself in a debate over the painfulness of paperwork. Begin by granting the patient's right to find the process tedious, then explain the value of the health history.

For a long-term solution to this complaint, the receptionist and dentist should review all hated paperwork and discuss how it could be streamlined. Many offices give patients a computerized copy of their health history form when they arrive for a visit. If the form is accurate, the patient simply signs and dates it.

Great answer "I know it seems tedious. We appreciate your help. We find that when we check with you about your health, we provide quality service that exactly matches your health needs." If the patient looks doubtful, you might add: "Your overall health influences dental treatment. For example, a patient with a heart condition may need premedication for a dental procedure. My own health status changed in the last few months, and it influenced how the doctor treated me."

"Why do I have to put down my age? My children don't even know how old I am!"

Possible answer "We do like to have complete records for our files. Most of our patients don't have any trouble answering these questions."

Comment Two guidelines to gain from this answer: Never give an answer that sounds as if you value records more than people, and never compare patients unless the comparison is favorable.

Great answer "You're wondering why we would need to know something that your own family doesn't? When I first started working here, I thought dentistry was pretty much the same for everyone. Was I wrong! There are hundreds of dental conditions that can affect our total health, and depending on our age, we are far more likely to be hit by some diseases than others. For example, mature adults are more at risk of oral cancer. So, your age is an important clue to helping the doctor diagnose some serious conditions." You might offer, "Would you be willing to put down an age range of ten years?"

Appointment Delays _____

"Why are you running behind?"

Possible answer "You know how Doctor is. Until everything is just right, he will not be happy. But let me go check for you."

Comment We must compliment this communicator on creativity. She was asked about a scheduling delay and bridged to the topic of quality care. But the underlying message is, "Yes, we're late. We're always late. Welcome to the practice where waiting is assured." This is not the image you want for your practice.

Possible answer "The doctor is tied up with a difficult case and will be with you shortly."

Comment Tell patients that the doctor finds cases difficult? It doesn't promote an image of clinical excellence.

Here are three tips for handling scheduling delays. First, tell patients about delays *before* they ask. They are usually nicer than if they already have engaged in foot-tapping and clock-watching. Second, if the delay in schedule is due to a dental emergency, say so. If you can briefly express sympathy for the emergency patient, so much the better. Third, tell patients that the delay will be slightly longer than the dentist says it will be. You may be able to exceed their revised expectations.

Great answer "Mrs. Smith, a dental emergency (or a special situation) with one of our patients has put the doctor's schedule about thirty minutes behind. That poor little girl! May I offer you a cup of coffee or a soft drink while you wait? Or would you like to use our phone to call someone about this unexpected delay?" You might add: "I did try to let you know about this in advance. You'll find a message from me on your answering machine when you get home."

"Why should I show up on time when I always have to wait?"

Comment This is a bigger problem than the communication style of the appointment coordinator. Solving it takes a concerted action by everyone in the practice. Practice management consultant Linda Miles recommends that if the doctor or hygienist is five minutes late, the receptionist is responsible for acknowledging such tardiness to the patient with an apology. If the doctor or hygienist is ten minutes late, he or she must go into the reception room and apologize in person to the waiting patient. With these policies in force, the office will never be more than nine-and-a-half minutes late.[3]

Great answer "It's very frustrating to have to wait. I give you my sincere apologies. I will let the doctor know that you are here right now. I will also find out when you will be seen. Then, you can decide what's best for you. I can offer you a cup of coffee or juice and the use of our phone if you need to call someone about this delay. Or we would certainly understand if you would prefer to reschedule."

Late Patient

"Sorry I'm late. You can still see me, right?"

Great answer "We were worried about you! We schedule appointments for the necessary time to provide quality service. In order to give you the quality care you deserve, we will have to reappoint you at a time convenient for you."

Great answer "I'm glad to see you! You're usually so prompt, I was getting a bit worried. I will let the doctor know you are here right now and see what your options are." After checking with the doctor, you might say, "Because we would never rush you and risk sacrificing the quality of your care, you have the choice of either receiving part of your treatment today, or reappointing at another time for all of your care at once."

Schedule Mix-up

"I know my appointment is for today." (The patient's appointment is for another day.)

Possible answer "Would it be convenient for you to come back at your scheduled appointment time? Or we could try to fit you in for at least part of your treatment."

Comment This answer assumes the patient is wrong about the appointment time. (Although that's usually the case, you can't say so.) If the practice takes responsibility for scheduling problems, patients are more likely to call in later and own up to their role in the mix-up. An excellent approach is to give patients several options for solving the situation. If patients are given choices, they are more often satisfied with solutions.

Great answer "This is so unfortunate! Our schedules don't match! I certainly apologize for the inconvenience. Let me see what our options are. Would you prefer to come in at (the time scheduled by the practice) or choose another time convenient for you, or have part of your treatment today?"

Afternoon Preschoolers _____

"Why can't I bring in my three-year-old at 4:00?"

Comment Many practices see preschoolers in the morning only because young children tend to be more rested and cooperative at that time. But with a growth in single-parent and dual-income families, this approach poses difficulties for some parents. Therefore, practices should give their appointment coordinators increased flexibility on this policy.

Great answer "It's difficult when the appointment times best for parents aren't the same as the times best for children. We all want a great visit for Elizabeth. If she comes in during the morning hours when our other preschoolers do, she will be more rested, alert, and ready for new experiences. Why don't we try a morning appointment and see how Elizabeth does?"

Three-month Recall _____

"I don't want the three-month recall appointment recommended by the hygienist. I'll come in six months. The hygienist must need to make another payment on her swimming pool."

Great answer "I will be happy to make a six-month appointment for you. But it sounds like the hygienist wasn't as clear as she meant to be about why a three-month recall visit is important for you, Mr. Anderson. It will help keep you in good health and prevent dental problems that can cause discomfort and added expense. Would you like to talk to the doctor about your recall schedule? Then if you still aren't sure about it, can I call you in two months to see how you are doing?"

Treatment Cancellation _____

"I need to cancel my appointment. My daughter told me I am too old to put that much money into one tooth."

Great answer "Mrs. Brown, I will cancel your appointment if that is what you prefer. But I won't be able to help worrying about you. This treatment is important to help you chew comfortably and gain full nutritional value from the food you eat. May I have your permission to schedule a consultation for you and your daughter to meet with the doctor and discuss your treatment?"

Questionable Emergency Patient _____

"I'm in pain and need to see the doctor right away. Noon? Noon isn't good; I can't miss 'All My Children.' No, 4:00 P.M. won't work either."

Comment Naturally, you see true dental emergencies immediately. First thing in the morning, the receptionist checks with clinical staff about preferred times for emergency visits. The receptionist asks emergency patients, "How quickly can you come to our office?" and schedules accordingly. If patients quibble about the convenience of emergency appointments, the receptionist can't question patient dedication or the seriousness of dental problems. But neither should she allow destruction of the carefully crafted daily schedule and risk inconveniencing other patients.

Great answer "I'm sorry, but noon and 4:00 P.M. are our only times available. I urge you to pick one. We would hate to see you even more uncomfortable tonight. But I'm sure you will make the right decision. Do you prefer one of those times, or do you want me to check on available times for tomorrow?"

Unwillingness to Appoint _____

"I don't know when a good appointment time would be. Can't I just call you?"

Great answer "Certainly. I'm going to note on my calendar that you plan to go ahead with the treatment, but you need to do some checking on times that would be most convenient for you. How about I call you within the next week or two to schedule the visit? Would your work or home number be best?"

Problem with Appointment Times _____

"Why don't you have an opening sooner than that (or at the time I prefer)?"

Great answer "It is certainly frustrating when the times you want are already taken. (Or: It is frustrating not to be able to have an appointment as promptly as you would like.) We sure appreciate patients like you who are dedicated about going ahead with the care they need. Let's schedule you so you have an appointed time. And may I put you on our special call list if an earlier appointment opens up?"

Practice management consultant Kathy Jameson recommends, "We reserve specific times of the day for this type of intricate and detailed procedure. In order for the doctor and the clinical team to give the necessary attention to you, we need to reserve special time. Tell me, are mornings or afternoons best for you?"[4]

"Why can't I just see another dentist in the practice to get in sooner?"

Possible answer   "If your dentist is in, you need to see him or her. Our other dentists will see you if your dentist isn't in town only as a courtesy to them or as an emergency."

Comment   Too much emphasis on serving the preferences of the doctors. As with all your answers, your focus must be on benefits to the patient.

Great answer   "Certainly it's frustrating not to have an appointment as soon as you would like. You are so dedicated, and we appreciate that. But the consistency of your care—being treated by someone who knows you well—is important to your comfort and your treatment. We would be more than happy to put you on our call list. But let's still schedule you so you do have an appointed time."

Appointment Confirmations _____

"Why do you always call me to remind me of my appointment? I've never forgotten."

Great answer   "You're right, you haven't. And we really appreciate it. I call everyone the day before the appointment as a matter of course. If we confirm the schedule that way, we do a better job of seeing patients on time. Plus you're one of the patients I enjoy chatting with. Do you really prefer I not call you to confirm next time?" (After this answer, few patients will tell you not to call.)

Phone Call for Dentist _____

"I want to talk directly to the doctor NOW." (patient telephone call)

Comment   The doctor is never "out," "busy," "on another line," or "unable to talk right now." Instead, the doctor is always involved in patient-oriented duties. For example, the doctor is "with a patient," "at a continuing education seminar," or "on an emergency call at the hospital."

Great answers   "Doctor Keenan is with a patient. How may I help you?" Or, "The doctor is with a patient. May I tell her what this is regarding?" Or, "Let me check for you. It may be five minutes. Would you prefer to hold, or shall I have him call you back?" And one more: "Of course you want to talk directly to the doctor, and you don't want to have to repeat yourself. Would you be willing to tell me the essentials of your condition so I can pass it on to the doctor? Then, he will review your chart to be able to give you better assistance when he returns your call."

Dentist Spouse

"What's it like working for your husband?"

Great answer "Wonderful! He does such excellent work, it's a pleasure to see the results of patient treatment. And he gets a chance to be impressed with me once in a while. Few couples have that opportunity."

Practice Growth

"The office has gotten so big, I'm just a number here. Why is everyone in such a hurry?"

Great answer "I'm so sorry! I would hate to think that we haven't let you know lately how much we value you as a patient. You're one of our favorites. We have had a number of new patients. I guess word has gotten out about our abilities. But we want patients like you who have been so loyal over the years to still feel comfortable with us. Anything in particular you would suggest? I'll take your ideas to our next staff meeting."

Parents in Treatment

"Why don't you let parents in the treatment room?"

Possible answer "Children behave best in the absence of their parents when there is a need for their total attention."

Comment Although this is an honest answer, it's not as positive as it could be. Some parents hear it as, "So this office thinks I'm a bad influence on my little Andy."

Dentists vary a great deal on their policies regarding parents in treatment. According to a 1980 survey by the Association of Pedodontic Diplomates, about 10 percent of pediatric dentists always allow parents into treatment, about 10 percent refuse under all circumstances, and the remaining 80 percent admit parents in selective cases.[5] The following answer discourages—but doesn't prohibit—parents in the treatment room.

Great answer "If you feel very strongly about it, we would be honored to have you. Let me tell you your options, and what seems to work best for most children. We all want a great visit for Andy. We find if we work with your child directly, we are able to build a rapport with him so he is comfortable with us. If Andy has a positive relationship with us right away, it gives him a better chance for a lifetime of good dental health."

Additional messages   "We can't compete with you, and we wouldn't try. We find when a child is in an unfamiliar setting, they look to the parent for rescue. If they are not rescued, they become upset with the parent—and then with us. We wouldn't want to see that happen with you and Andy."

"Do you know what research shows is one of the biggest differences between adults who have good dental health and adults who don't? Whether that adult had a good relationship with a dentist as a child. That's why building rapport with Andy as quickly as possible is so important."

Parent Management Tips

- Recognize that your office differs from parental expectations. For example, parents do not send children alone into treatment in a pediatrician's office. Parents typically accompany their children into health-care settings and are expected to physically assist with care.

- Recognize that when a parent watches you relate effectively to a child, it's an excellent marketing opportunity for your practice.

- Mail parent education materials in advance of first visits on how to prepare children for dental treatment. This will prevent parents from giving negative reassurance ("I won't let the doctor hurt you") or making threats ("If you don't brush, I'm going to tell the dentist").

- When parents arrive for their child's visit, educate them in their role as "silent partner." Let them know what is—and isn't—helpful to their child.

- Minimize parental involvement by saying, "Why don't you come back and help us get Jennifer settled, then relax in reception if you like." Or, you might say, "Allow us to get Jennifer settled, then feel free to come back and check on her as often as you like."

- If a parent comes back to treatment, put the parent's chair out of the child's line of sight and as far away from the action as possible. Or don't provide a chair and invite the parent to watch from the doorway.

- Don't leave all your interesting magazines in reception. Have some in the treatment room to give parents something to read during procedures.

- One enterprising dental office tells parents, "You deserve a treat. Here's a beeper and a coupon for cappuccino at the cafe across the street. We'll beep you if we need you." The dentist notes that this approach saves far more in time than it costs in coffee.

Skill Summary

- When a patient is anxious, upset, or confused, begin your answer with an acknowledgment of the patient's point of view. If possible, give the patient a choice between several options for solving the situation.

- Remember to say "thank you" to the patients who arrive on time, fill out forms carefully, pay promptly, refer other patients to your practice, and the like.

- Look for opportunities to communicate the following messages:

  - The dental care you will receive today is precisely matched to your medical and dental health needs.

  - This practice prides itself on providing the highest quality of care possible. It's a pleasure for me to see the results of patient treatment.

  - The continuity of your care—being treated by someone who knows you well—is important to your comfort and your health.

  - You are very wise to seek regular dental treatment. It's the best way to protect your health and your pocketbook.

  - We value every one of our patients—but you are one of our favorites.

References

1. Zunin L, Zunin N. Contact: The First Four Minutes. New York: Ballantine Books; 1972.

2. Hastorf A, Schneider DJ, Ellsworth P. Person Perception, ed 2. Reading, MA: Addison-Wesley Publications; 1979.

3. Miles LL. Practice Dynamics. Tulsa, OK: Pennwell Publishing Company; 1986:60.

4. Jameson C. Great Communication = Great Production. Tulsa, OK: Pennwell Publishing Company; 1994:180.

5. Rayman MS. Parent observation. CDA Journal 1987;August: 20–24.

Communication Goals for the Dental Team

"Problems are opportunities in work clothes."

—Henry Kaiser

Imagine this situation: You are having a terrible day. Your practice schedule is packed with patients from hell. You stay late for an emergency patient, which makes you late picking up your son from soccer practice. You stop at the dry cleaners and manage to lock your keys (all your keys) in the car.

Tired and cranky, you and your son trudge home, hoping someone will be there. You pound on the locked door of your house; no one is home. Suddenly you notice an odd flickering light through a window on the upper floor.

Some possibilities run through your mind. It could be a faulty light fixture, which means you need to check the bulb and electrical outlet. It could be a small fire, which means you may need to get a fire extinguisher or call the fire department. But before you can fix the problem—or even discover what the problem is—you need an extra set of house keys.

Good communication is the key to good patient relationships. Anticipating tough questions and planning how to manage them is knowing where the extra keys are. The theme of this book is not to guarantee that you will never be locked out of a patient's mind, heart, or relationship. The theme is to think about that possibility in advance so you have an extra set of keys—communication skills that can unlock the doors to patient understanding and treatment acceptance.

When you have effective communication with patients, they are more likely to understand and agree with treatment recommendations. They are more likely to be comfortable during treatment, comply with post-treatment instructions, and recuperate more quickly. They are more likely to refer other patients to your practice, pay their bills on time, and be satisfied with their dental care. May the benefits of good communication be yours. And may you always carry an extra set of keys.

Appointment Coordinator

Communication Job Description

- Make everyone feel welcome, at home, warm, important.
- Give each patient a sense of quality and thoroughness in their care.
- Let the patient know that the practice provides the best possible care.
- Achieve a smile from the patient immediately.
- Answer questions in a knowledgeable way.
- Make patients feel good about choosing the practice.
- Greet each patient by name.
- Inform patients of any necessary waiting time.
- Check on new information for patient records.

Business Manager

Communication Job Description

- Help patients see their time and money as an investment to achieve their personal goals of keeping their teeth for a lifetime.
- Help patients receive the maximum possible insurance benefits.
- Help patients feel comfortable with their financial arrangements.
- Keep patients from losing sight of the fact that they must make a commitment to their health.
- Relate to patients the true value of the services offered.
- Explain insurance benefits so patients understand both their coverage and their responsibilities.
- Be up-front and honest with patients about costs; the goal is "No surprises."
- Help patients afford good dental care.
- Make financial complications obsolete.

Dental Assistant

Communication Job Description

- Learn as much as possible about every new patient.
- Get to know each patient's personality, wants, and values.
- Help each patient understand his or her dental needs.
- Prepare each new patient to accept a complete exam and necessary X-rays.
- Let every patient know that the dental team is there to help meet his or her dental goals in terms of health, function, and appearance.
- Help each patient feel comfortable and relaxed.
- Show a sincere interest in the patient's oral health.
- Reinforce the benefits of treatment and the disadvantages of no treatment.
- Be sure each patient understands the cost, time, and payment method for the treatment.

Dental Hygienist

Communication Job Description

- Help patients understand the importance of protecting their long-term oral health.
- Make visits comfortable and enjoyable for patients so they want to return.
- Treat each patient as an individual by getting to know his or her dental values, attitudes, and knowledge level.
- Let each patient know in a nonjudgmental way the effectiveness of his or her home-care habits.
- Provide oral health education in understandable and motivating ways.
- Reinforce the benefits of treatment and the disadvantages of no treatment.
- Communicate a message of quality preventive care to every patient.
- Assist the dentist with community outreach projects related to preventive dentistry.

Dentist

Communication Job Description

- Carefully prepare the dental team to respond positively to patient concerns.
- Support the dental team in their communication with patients.
- Keep patients involved in their commitment to oral and total health.
- Confirm patient understanding of the true value of the service offered.
- Present clear, concise treatment plans.
- Listen well and adapt communication to each patient's point of view.
- Help each patient feel comfortable as a member of the practice family.
- Build patient trust in the practice and dental team.

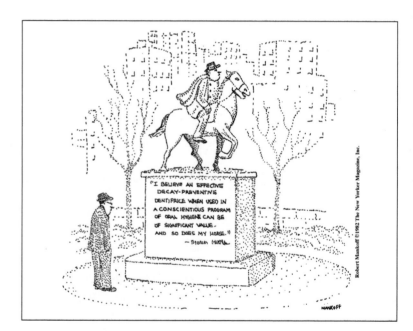

Index